How to Keep or Regain Health in Times of Worldwide Pollution

Showing different methods and therapies such as homeopathy and Chinese medicine to cope with toxins aquired from infections and environment in comparison to orthodox medical treatment

by Ilse G. Knauf MD

How to keep or regain health in times of worldwide pollution

by Ilse G. Knauf MD

Table of contents

Foreword   page 9

Introduction   page 11

General considerations on cancer and its
causing agents   page 12

The chronic fatigue syndrome   page 18

Viruses, bacteria and a fungus that had been
linked to this syndrome   page 18

Epstein Barr Virus   page 18

Cytomegalo virus   page 20

Herpes 6 virus   page 22

The Coxsackie virus group   page 23

Borrelia Burgdorferi   page 24

Chlamydia pneumoniae   page 28

Candida albicans   page 30

The cycle of energy production
The role of mitochondria   page 32

The role of cholesterol in our metabolism   page 34

More risk factors for the development of
atherosclerosis   page 37
Homocystein
Dimethylargenine
C-reactive protein
Lipoprotein a

Factors counteracting degenerative diseases   page 40
Anthocyanins
The carotinoids
Huperzine A
The salvestrols and resveratrol
Modified citrus pectin
S adenosyl methionine

The dangers of glycation   page 43

The influence of radioactivity on our
immune-system   page 45
Radioactive Thorium   page 45
Iodine   page 46
Caesium   page 47
Strontium   page 48

Consequences of toxic environment and
faulty behaviour   page 49

General considerations on autoimmune
processes   page 53

General considerations on allergies   page 54

Ways of cleansing the body by eliminating foci
or toxic tooth fillings   page 56

Regaining health by proper nutrition   page 57

General considerations on environmental
conditions   page 59

Toxic heavy metals   page 61
Cadmium   page 61
Lead   page 62
Mercury   page 64
Chelating agents to remove toxic heavy
metals   page 65
Problems related to platinum and worldwide
traffic   page 68

Breathing and exercise   page 70

Antioxidants and nutritional balance   page 71

Problems with asbestos   page 75

The ozone dilemma   page 76

General considerations on fasting   page 78

The importance of the intestinal flora for
the whole system   page 80

How to clean the body by fasting   page 86

Treatment with homeopathy   page 92

The basics of Chinese medicine   page 97

The function of the yin organs   page 98

The meridians   page 99

Energy flow and psychosomatic illness   page 101

Making the energy field visible   page 104

Different forms of psychotherapy   page 107

Comparing the orthodox approach with Chinese therapies   page 109

Mistakes we will have to pay for   page 111

How nutrition can be improved   page 113

Allergies, incompatibilities and homeopathy   page 116

Miasma and homeopathic therapy   page 118

Attention Deficit Hyperactivity Syndrome   page 121

Autoimmune diseases with possible ways
of treatment   page 123

Comparison between homeopathy and
Chinese medicine   page 126

Different diseases and comparison of
treatment (in alphabetical order)   page 127
Acne and other skin diseases   page 127

Allergies   page 129

Atherosclerosis   page 132

Arthritis   page 136
Asthma and related problems   page 140

Baldness and hair loss   page 144

Cancer development   page 147

Cardiologic problems   page 154

Chronic inflammation of the bowel   page 156

Diabetes   page 159

Gout as a result of elevated uric acid   page 161

Hypertension as a risk factor   page 164

Liver problems   page 167

Lung problems   page 174
Menstrual imbalances and other
gynaecological problems   page 176

Multiple sclerosis   page 179

Osteoporosis and osteomalacia   page 181

Parkinson's disease   page 184

Pharyngitis   page 186

Sinusitis   page 187

Chinese herbs for medicinal use   page 190
(in alphabetical order)

Chinese formulas in detail   page 220

List of important homeopathic remedies   page 228

Selected homeopathic remedies for
special indications   page 234

Recipes for special juices   page 240

Acai berries and Grapefruit juice   page 241
(showing interactions with chemical
medication)

Foreword

This book has been written after more than 30 years of work as a general practitioner and as a gynecologist in hospitals and private practice, and it is a summary of the experiences I had with my patients while treating them with different approaches to health problems.

After passing through the conventional medical school in Germany I came into contact with various ways of treatment, which besides the orthodox way comprises classic homeopathy, chiropractic treatment, nutritional science, psychotherapy and Chinese medicine. They all have a right in their own way, and together give you a means to select the appropriate complementary method, especially when you have come to a limit with the conventional approach to disease. This was often the case with all sorts of allergies, autoimmune illness and most of the chronic degenerative forms of diseases, which are so frequent in our highly civilized and sterilized environment.

When I lived in America and learned more about nutritional science, chiropractic treatment and psychotherapy, I found it was highly complementary to the European way of classic homeopathy and orthodox medicine that I had known until then. Everything could be integrated into a holistic approach to health management, and together all those methods yielded the best results.

When I try to explain the principles of Chinese medicine in this book, it is meant to show the way of thinking of this old culture, which is so completely contrary to our western approach to health issues, but the section on herbal medicine would not make sense without a few explanations of that kind.

Another aim of this book is to give some basic knowledge about important diseases, and to compare the different ways of treatment. That comprises Chinese medicine as well as homeopathic remedies and methods of cleansing the organism with fasting, proper nutrition and breathing.
Certainly the orthodox way of treatment will be mentioned as well, and a little biochemistry and genetics will be interspersed to show how sophisticated the metabolism of our body is.
But the readers who are not interested in medical or biochemical details can skip those parts and still will be able to follow up on the contents of the therapeutic recommendations and comparison of the different methods.

When I talk about different ways of psychotherapy it shows my personal opinions concerning that topic, and you can come to different conclusions, but everything I say came out of the experience with patients, though it may not be the currently held opinion of colleagues who work in that field.
The Chinese and homeopathic sections at the end of this book show a survey on some of the most important remedies used in that field, and give recommendations for treatment of specific illnesses such as allergies, arthritis, sinusitis and so on.

All this is not meant as an encouragement for self-treatment, but intends to show different possibilities that exist, so everyone can find the practitioner who is an expert in one or several of the fields mentioned in this book.

Introduction

Climate change and worldwide pollution have turned out to be the greatest challenge of our time, and there is an ever-increasing gap between the richer northern countries and the poorer south. The problem the rich countries will have to face with an aging population is that with more sick people they may not be able to take care of them properly. Illnesses, chronic in character, pose many problems and cost a lot of resources.

Diabetes and cancer rates do not seem to decline in spite of intense research done for that purpose, so we want to follow up on the question of different possibilities in terms of prophylaxis and treatment that can be called complementary, in comparison with orthodox medical regimens.

In the course of this book I will try to point out diverse approaches to prominent ailments of our time, for instance how the Chinese point of view and the homeopathic form of treatment see a problem and try to cope with it, compared to the orthodox way.

All types of toxins from within and without surround us, and nobody really knows if he is still healthy, or if a time bomb is already ticking in his body that will become manifest later in his life by creating some illness like cancer, diabetes or Parkinson's disease.

As the author of this book worked as a gynaecologist and as a general practitioner, and also for several years in a private health clinic, the experience with patients fasting and being treated with herbal remedies will be given some space.

All this has taken place in Europe, working with patients from different countries, but most of the cases described here could have happened anywhere in the world.

We will try to look not only at the symptoms on the surface, but to find the roots of illnesses and show how the worst can be prevented by different eating habits or a change in the way of thinking. When in the course of this book treatments are described it goes without saying that I had a team working with me on our patients, and that is why I from now on refer to 'we' in the context of this book.

We will start with the one illness that causes the most anxiety, and that is cancer. Trying to point out risk factors first and showing in later chapters things that can be done as prophylaxis or complementary treatment, while the orthodox medical way will be mentioned too.

General considerations on Cancer and its causing agents

- Toxic substances
- Radioactivity
- Certain viruses
- Oxygen deficiency
- Depression of the immune system through stress

It has been known for a long time that the development of cancer can take up to one third of the lifetime of an individual. It depends on several factors, such as the amount of toxic substances that have been ingested and the resistance of the respective person or animal.

If a human has been afflicted with noxious chemicals, or with radioactive particles, as has been the case after nuclear disasters, it could take quite a number of years till a cancer is manifested.

Even viruses can be carcinogenic, that means being able to cause cancer. It was known for quite a while that the EBV (Epstein Barr Virus) had been present in Burkitt lymphomas, a malignant growth of the lymphatic system.

In the 1970's it was found that certain members of the HPV group (Human Papilloma Virus) were causative in almost 100% of cervix carcinomas.

In the field of gynaecology the routine with the Pap smear has brought some relief. The alterations of the surface cells of the cervix uteri can be detected fairly early with that method, so that survival rates for this tumour could be largely increased.

Unfortunately people in risk groups are underrepresented when it comes to taking advantage of the tests; therefore we still have casualties due to this sort of cancer.

The vaccination for certain aggressive viruses of that group has now been available for a number of years, and it will hopefully yield another decrease in the manifestation of that disease.

There are other tumours that cannot so easily be detected as for instance pancreatic cancer, because this organ is not so easily accessible.

Then there are the problems with impaired respiration, which are frequently occurring with allergic illnesses such as asthma or chronic pulmonary disease such as asbestosis, leading to lack of oxygen in tissues. This makes them more vulnerable to cell alterations, and can end up in tumour growth.

All that is true, but also the human psyche seems to play an important role in the manifestation of all major diseases.

It was found that psycho-traumatic incidents can weaken the immune system, as for instance the loss of a beloved family member, and we had quite a number of patients who had a carcinoma become manifest after the death of a child or a partner.

We call that stress, and there is general agreement on the point that stress is crucial for a majority of illnesses, but what exactly happens in our body when some kind of psycho-trauma takes place?

To understand that we have to take a closer look at our neuro-endocrine system, that means the connection between our nerve system and our hormonal balance.

The hormones in our body are ruled by the pituitary gland; this is what we learned in medical school, but who rules the pituitary? The answer is that the hypothalamus does, and that is a part of our brain, which is in connection with all the other parts of our brain, especially the limbic system. We can see that the limbic system is the centre for our emotional life, in which the hypothalamus plays a major role. Meaning our emotions influence the hypothalamus, which in turn produces the releasing hormones. The pituitary gland puts the information through to the other hormonal glands such as the thyroid, the gonads and what is most important in a stress situation to the adrenals via the adrenocorticotropic hormone. Thus signalling for the adrenal cortex to produce mineralocorticoids and glucocortioids, which among other things raise blood sugar levels and slow down digestion.

But most important is the production of epinephrine (adrenaline), which is produced in the adrenal medulla under the influence of the sympathetic part of the autonomous nerve system as a stress reaction. Besides elevating our heart rate and blood pressure it enhances memories of past traumatic events, thus causing fear. When we consider all that, it becomes quite clear why the two most important stress hormones, adrenaline and cortisole, which are produced under the influence of our emotions, surge to high levels in case of an emergency.

In that case the essential goal will be to survive, and it is the task of our autonomous nerve system to take care of that. This system is divided into two parts, the sympathetic and the parasympathetic. While the sympathetic has to see that we survive in case of danger, the other part, the parasympathetic, has to provide peace and nourishment. When we have to fight or flee, nourishment is no longer important, because life has to be saved first, but after that episode the system has to be brought back to its normal peace. The sympathetic system can save our life by quickly activating our alertness and muscular strength, but this is not meant to last for a long time; when the danger is gone everything is supposed to go back to normal such as our heart rate or our blood pressure. That means the hormones that grant our survival in case of an emergency, causing our blood pressure and heart rate to go up in order to be able to create maximum strength for fight or flight, should come back to a lower level when that danger is gone.

Otherwise we stay in a state of emergency, though actually the danger that threatened us no longer exists. The consequence of a sympathetic overhang can be high blood pressure and a rapid heart rate, together with elevated blood sugar levels, which may stay that way permanently, thus leaving our system as though under constant stress. This becomes quite hazardous, as the vital functions of getting proper nutrition and oxygen for our cells suffer that way, and what is most important, our immune system will not be able to fulfil its normal function, as elevated cortisole levels interfere with the production and function of immune competent cells, such as B and T-Lymphocytes.

It also slows down the healing of wounds and impedes the metabolism of our bones. Those facts may be the crucial point for the development of cancer or other severe illnesses such as osteoporosis and many others.

What causes our body to live under conditions that had been appropriate for an acute situation, but turn out to be detrimental for our normal life? Obviously the memories of dangerous situations that caused fear can be stored in our mind, some of them are conscious and others are unconscious. They may have happened at an early age that we do not remember actively, but our unconscious mind has stored them like the images on a film. If they were threatening and are being reactivated, we fall back into the pattern that once was needed for a dangerous situation, but now is no longer adequate. The trigger for such a situation can be anything in the present that brings back the memory, and causes the same fight or flight reactions that then had been appropriate. But now they are no longer, because we are no longer in danger.

If for instance there had been an accident, where the person almost drowned, it can happen that every contact with water brings back those memories of life threatening peril, and even looking at a harmless pond can trigger that fearful reaction. What can be done to stop those vicious cycles? The solution would be to make this trigger mechanism ineffective by taking the charge out of those old images on the film of our memory, and thus keeping them from reactivating the neuro-hormonal responses that once were necessary to survive in an emergency situation.

Now they make our life a misery by forcing us to live under constant circumstances of stress, thus squandering our energies unnecessarily, deprive our whole system of rest and recreation, and weaken our immune system. This can lead to all sorts of illnesses including allergies and tumours.

Now the crucial point remains as how to take the charge, which creates tension, out of those old traumatic memories. As we want to stop the vicious cycle that ever and again pulls us back into reactions, which are no longer appropriate, but can create chronic illness. Many different answers have been given to that question, and we will try to sort them out in the course of this book when we speak about different ways of psychotherapy.

Another problem has been intriguing us for quite a while, as so many people complain about being tired most of the time. Probably also this phenomenon is closely linked to our emotions and immune system, as feelings of fear and rejection can start vicious cycles affecting and weakening the whole system. But we will have to look at all the details to find out what role some agents play in connection with the above mentioned facts.

The Chronic Fatigue Syndrome

Viruses and bacteria that had been linked to that syndrome

- Epstein-Barr virus
- Cytomegalo virus
- Herpes- 6 virus
- The Coxsackie virus group
- Borrelia Burgdorferi
- Chlamydia pneumoniae
- Candida albicans

Epstein-Barr virus

The number of patients feeling exhausted most of the time has increased on a large scale, and therefore this syndrome, which is a collection of symptoms, has been named Chronic Fatigue Syndrome or CFS. As mostly no substantial derangements could be found in laboratory tests, it was suspected that viruses were the reason, why people had lost so much of their energy, and therefore certain viruses got under suspicion.

The first one was the Epstein Barr Virus (EBV), as in quite a number of patients antibodies against that virus could be found, and so it was speculated that a reactivation of this virus might be the reason for CFS. Normally the EBV is the active agent in infectious mononucleosis, a disease that mostly takes place in teenage years and causes lymph node swellings and a sore throat besides feeling tired and sick.

That virus belongs to the herpes group, meaning it is a persistent virus, as all the members of that group are, and it will stay with you for the rest of your life.

More than 90% of the population worldwide have sometime in their life contact with the EBV, therefore the finding of antibodies does not have to mean that this is the reason for CFS. A closer look at the constellation of antibodies may give a clue if reactivation has really taken place, as there are different sorts of antibodies in the early and the late phases of a disease. But it may be that in spite of reactivation it is not the only reason for existing ailments, though it could have contributed to the state of fatigue.

Every active virus costs the host a lot of energy, because it forces the organism, it has befallen, to replicate its own genetic material, which can be DNA or RNA.

In case EBV has been involved in an illness we are confronted with the problem that no close correlation exists between the amounts of antibodies, found in a blood sample, and the severity of the disease. That means, though there are only a few antibodies in the blood of the host, the patient can have a severe form of EBV illness.

But we have known for a long time that the microbe is not the most important thing to make a patient sick, but the terrain on which it can grow, as the French physiologist Claude Bernard had found out more than a hundred years ago, when he said " Le microbe c'est rien, le milieu c'est tout."

That means if an organism is weakened in any way by stress or toxins, a virus can gain a lot of space and replicate at a fast rate, because the resistance of the host is low at that point.

That often happens with the EBV, it can start making symptoms, whenever the host organism comes under stress and is weakened. This makes sense when we consider the connection between stress and the immune system. But soon other viruses came into focus, which were held responsible for causing fatigue.

Cytomegalo virus

The next one was the Cytomegalo virus that was accused of at least contributing to the CFS. This virus also belongs to the herpes family, and causes similar ailments as EBV, but it mostly goes along with minor symptoms, and therefore may not be detected so soon. But it can also be aggressive, and having an affinity to the kidneys it can do a lot of harm to that organ.

In case someone gets a kidney transplant, which was infected with that virus it can run riot in the recipient's body, then being in a state of immune suppression, in order to prevent the rejection of the foreign organ. Even under normal circumstances this virus can be reactivated and contribute to a state of ill health, if the person is suffering from stress or toxins.

But also that virus did not qualify as sole culprit for the CFS, because here also a lot of conditioning factors have to be present to create the fatigue. Nevertheless the correlation between antibody titres, which measure the amount of antibodies being found in the blood of the patient, and the illness seems to be more reliable than in EBV cases.

Blood tests nowadays are being done with an ELISA test, i.e. enzyme-linked immune sorbent assay, out of the patient's serum, and have totally replaced former laboratory tests. As viruses do not respond to antibiotic therapy, great efforts had been undertaken to find a possibility to help those patients. In case of this virus the substance Gancyclovir is used as virostatic treatment, that way the DNA replication of the virus is inhibited, but it never disappears completely.

Therefore it seems important to tell people how an infection can be prevented, as this virus can be transmitted sexually or through blood or body fluids. Frequent washing of hands, especially before eating with bare fingers is essential, and otherwise safer sex is as important as in the prevention of HIV infection, the human immune deficiency virus, which can cause AIDS. Also in the prevention of B-type hepatitis and many other diseases people should not be as careless as they may have been in former times.

The combination of two viruses, such as Cytomegalo and HIV, is extremely dangerous and can lead to severe symptoms of Cytomegalo infection with organ damage.

The treatment of viral diseases with homoeopathy or Chinese medicine will be described in a later chapter, and stress management is equally important

Herpes-6 virus

Then the next virus, which also belongs to the herpes group, got into focus, and that was the Herpes-6 virus, which was discovered in 1986 in the United States. It can cause lympho-reticular disorders befalling T-lymphocytes. It is also one of the eight members of the human herpes family and there are two different types A and B of that virus. The latter type causes the disease Roseola infantum, also called Exanthema subitum or sixth disease, it affects babies and young infants and goes along with raised red skin and fever that can last for several days. Sometimes it can be confused with measles or rubella, and in spite of the possibility of high fever infants tend to recover fully. The symptoms in this case mostly disappear without any treatment, but the virus can stay dormant for a long time, and it can be reactivated later in life under stress conditions, and then it may cause neurological symptoms, as well as a form of mononucleosis.

In this it is similar to the Varicella-Zoster virus, which causes chickenpox in young individuals beginning with a rash on the head and body and later on arms and legs.

As it is an airborne disease, it is very contagious when the virus particles are inhalded someone has spread by coughing or sneezing. This virus can stay dormant in the nervous system in the dorsal ganglia or the trigeminus ganglion and can later be reactivated as shingles (Herpes zoster).

In both cases patients under chemotherapy or immune suppression as well as AIDS patients are prone to suffer from a reactivation, as they have a compromised immune system.

For the herpes-6 virus Gancyclovir as virostatic treatment could be used too, especially for patients waiting for bone marrow transplant. This may be necessary for the treatment of leukaemia after chemotherapy and radiation, when the original marrow has to be destroyed.

The virostatic agents Acyclovir or Famacyclovir can be used for the treatment of the Varicella-zoster virus, especially for complications such as herpes zoster ophthalmicus, affecting the eye, or myelitis, affecting the spinal cord. The homeopathic therapy for that disease will be presented later, it basically tries to strengthen the immune system.

We have seen that several factors have to be present to create severe symptoms and cause chronic fatigue, those can be radiation, toxins, stress, or co-infection with HIV or other agents.

Coxsackie B virus

This was not the last virus that got under suspicion, the next was the Coxsackie B virus family, belonging to the Entero-viruses.

The Entero-virus family consists of 5 members, being slightly different from one another, but they all are mostly transmitted orally or with food.

Evidence was found that this virus group might cause T-cell mediated autoimmune destruction of pancreatic beta cells. It can initiate an inflammation of the islets of Langerhans, which produce insulin, and thus lead to type1 diabetes. We will be occupied with the different forms of diabetes and their treatment later.

First we have to explain what the expression T-cell mediated means, because it is a phenomenon that occurs almost universally in the development of autoimmune diseases. T-cells belong to the lymphocyte family, T standing for thymus, as they are activated in that organ, they are active immune cells, which can be divided into several sub groups. T-cells can initiate an autoimmune process directly without the mediation of antibodies, in contrast to allergies, where immune globulins, mostly of the E-type, start the immune reaction. We will talk about those T-cells cells later in more detail, because they also play an important role in the development or prevention of cancer.

The Coxsackie B group, besides being accused of initiating autoimmune processes, can cause aseptic meningitis, which is an inflammation in the brain without bacteria. Other disturbances of the central nervous system such as encephalitis, can also occur.

Besides that there have been numerous cases of myocarditis (inflammtion of the heart), which could result in heart failure and even death, as a consequence of Coxsackie B virus infection. But also in those cases a lowered immune resistance is usually the cause of the complications mentioned here.

Borrelia

Not only viruses were accused of causing CFS, but there were also bacteria that had led to cases of chronic illness with fatigue, such as Lyme disease. It was named after a town in Connecticut, New England, because the agent causing the disease, Borrelia Burgdorferi, was first described there. This agent is transmitted by different sorts of ticks such as Ixodes ricinus, which have the Borreliae in their stomachs and spit them out in the course of blood sucking.

A number of cases had been found in Connecticut producing symptoms that included fatigue, joint pain, headaches, fever and nausea. They started mostly with skin symptoms, such as a red ring surrounding the former insect sting. As the ring extends on the outside, it gets paler in the centre. This bacterium, Borrelia, is transmitted to the host through ticks during their development cycle.

The female tick lays thousands of eggs and the hatching larvae feed mostly on the blood of little insectivores for several days. Then they develop into the next stage, which is called nymphs, before they reach the final stage of adult ticks.

The infection of humans can take place with nymphs or adult insects that hover on high grass or small shrubs and drop when a potential victim passes by. In the course of bloodsucking the bacterium is transmitted to an animal or human, but this does not happen immediately. It takes the tick several hours to transport the Borrelia out of its stomach and spit it into the wound, together with secretions that keep the blood of the host from clotting.

Therefore it is essential to get rid of the tick as soon as possible. The later stages of the insect live normally in small rodents such as mice or rabbits. Even deer may be the victims or the hunters of small rodents like cats and dogs.

The bacterium has the form of a corkscrew and is related to an agent called Treponema pallidum, by which syphilis is transmitted in humans. This disease was much feared in former times when it occurred in Europe after Columbus had detected the New World and had brought it with him. In the era, when no antibiotics were available, this disease was life-threatening, as it could cause encephalitis or myelopathy of the dorsal columns of the spinal cord.

Lyme disease on the other hand can cause all kinds of ailments from arthritic pain to central-nervous or heart symptoms.

If during the first few weeks the illness goes unnoticed, and is not treated with antibiotics, it becomes more and more difficult to get rid of the agent.

Then Borrelia is able to penetrate into fibrous tissue cells and cannot be reached so easily by antibiotics, so that the disease can become chronic. Lyme disease can mimic all kinds of diseases and therefore can for a long time be overlooked.

Many people who like to spend much of their time outdoors became victims of ticks that dropped on legs or feet of humans who passed the bushes or shrubs where the ticks were hovering. The initial sting cannot be felt, and so many hours could elapse before the victim would realize that it had been stung.

We had also a number of patients who could not recall any tick bite, and later were found with antibodies against Borrelia, because they showed suspicious symptoms.

As only a small number of ticks are infested with the agent, many people did not think of the possibility that a dangerous bacterium could have entered their body, even if they tick bite could be remembered. Therefore antibody testing should be carried out in case ailments such as joint pains with swelling occur, especially if the knee is concerned.

Borrelia Burgdorferi is endemic in the United States, but there are two more types of Borrelia in Europe, namely B. Garinii and B. Afzelii, which are slightly different in their antigen pattern and the symptoms they cause. All the trials with vaccines have not been successful, as they did not cover the antigens of all the different types.

We had quite a number of cases, where Lyme disease became chronic and the patients suffered from pain all over the body accompanied by great fatigue despite the application of antibiotics, which obviously had been given too late. In those cases we treated our patients with a combination of the Borrelia nosode and cleansing remedies, which will be explained later.

One case of Lyme disease, which was quite spectacular, is worth mentioning, because the testing for antibodies had twice been negative, before it finally, after several months became positive. The young patient had been pregnant and during that time developed more and more symptoms that could be consistent with Lyme disease. She got joint swelling of her left knee and became so dizzy that she easily lost her balance, and gradually could not walk any more without being steadied by a second person or clinging to an object.

After the delivery of the baby we made another test, because the suspicion had arisen that the pregnancy might have interfered with the building of antibodies. The whole immune system during pregnancy has to show some immune tolerance towards the baby, in order not to endanger the child and reject it as foreign, as only half of the genes originate in his mother. The other part of the baby's genes, originating in his father, could otherwise be considered as alien, and rejected by the maternal immune system.

In this case the antibody test had probably been negative, because of the maternal immune tolerance during pregnancy, which also kept the mother from building antibodies against the Borrelia agent. Finally, after the baby had been delivered, the test became positive.

The mother who by then was hardly able to walk, as her sense for balance had suffered badly, made a full recovery with the help of homeopathic medication. Even the child needed some assistance, as it had been sick all the time with rhinitis and catarrh. The therapy for mother and child then consisted of homeopathic remedies with nosodes, after a former antibiotic regimen had not brought the desired success. This sort of therapy will be explained later in detail

Chlamydia pneumoniae

The last bacterium, we want to consider, is very special, as it is quite tiny, and was in the beginning taken for a virus. This agent is called Chlamydia pneumoniae, and is not to be confused with Chlamydia trachomatis. That latter agent is mostly sexually transmitted and leads to an inflammation of the cervix uteri and the Fallopian tubes and can end up in chronic Pelvic Inflammatory Disease with consecutive sterility in women and in epididymitis (inflammation) in men. The epididymis is a curved structure in the back of the testicle in which sperm is matured and stored.
Chlamydia trachomatis can also cause conjunctivitis and finally blindness or initiate reactive arthritis in the body called Reiter's syndrome with arthritis, conjunctivitis and

urethritis. Furthermore it can be transmitted from mother to child in the course of vaginal birth.

Overall it is one of the major causes for blindness in third world countries, where hygiene conditions are not good and a prophylactic eye therapy after birth is not given.

The Chlamydia pneumoniae bacterium on the other hand, had only been discovered in the 1980's and is transmitted by aerosols from infected people who cough and sneeze, in the same way as most viruses causing catarrhs are transmitted.

This Chlamydia pneumoniae virus turned out to be quite nasty, as it can cause illnesses of various kinds, and like the other Chlamydia it has a complicated life cycle in the cells of the host, as it cannot create energy of its own, but it sucks energy from the infected cells.

It can lead to pharyngitis, (that is inflammation of the throat,) bronchitis, pneumonia, and it can cause asthma symptoms and swelling of cervical lymph nodes.

It has also been accused of being a causing agent for multiple sclerosis, an autoimmune disease that befalls nerve tissue.

The treatment with the macrolide antibiotic Azithromycin is recommended, but it does not always eliminate the bacterium. We have seen patients, where the infection persisted for years in spite of treatment with different antibiotics, and asthmatic symptoms were really severe besides the patients' suffering from swelling of their lymph nodes and from total fatigue.

But also in those cases it was the unhealthy terrain that created the severe cases. It is a weakened immune resistance that enables the bacterium to further replicate and stay in lymphatic tissue for a long time.

With the approach of cleansing the body with herbal medicine, and giving support with the respective nosodes and homeopathic or Chinese herbal treatment, most patients, even with severe symptoms, could recover. Sometimes it took a very long time, that means several years, until the immune system of the host could get rid of that agent.

It turned out that one Chinese herb was very good in that context, and that was Artemisia annua, a remedy used in recent years mostly to combat malaria.

Because of similarities such as the intracellular growth of the malaria plasmodium and the Chlamydia, we started using that plant for our patients, and found it to be quite helpful.

Candida albicans

One more agent to disturb the body harmony is worth mentioning, and that is Candida albicans. It is a diploid fungus, appearing as yeast and as filamentous cells, called hyphal formation, when it gets invasive into certain tissues. It has been held responsible for quite a number of ailments, for instance opportunistic infections of the mouth and gastro-intestinal tract or genito-urinary system, as well as for diaper rash in infants. Other skin problems because of candida are frequent in diabetics or immune incompetent patients. The agent is normally living as a harmless saprophyte in the bowels of most humans, without causing major harm. But in the course of excessive use of antibiotics and faulty nutrition with an overload of sugar or the use of oral contraceptives it could start growing at a faster rate because of the change in terrain conditions.

As synthetic hormones alter the normal steady state in the female genital tract, and antibiotics do the same in the bowels, the Candida fungus can grow more rapidly under the changed conditions. Then it leads to ailments such as vaginitis with intense itching, or a bloated abdomen because of gas produced by the fungus out of carbohydrates.

Frequently the rapid overgrowth of those tissues with Candida is accompanied by a feeling of weakness and fatigue. But in most cases the terrain can be restored by treating the deranged bowel flora with probiotics such as acidophilus cultures and homeopathic therapy with nosodes, as will be described later.

Changing eating habits also helps a great deal to make the ailments subside, as especially sugar enhances the growth of Candida. The orthodox therapy with fungistatic medication such as fluconazole mostly gives only temporary relief. After a few weeks the Candida normally tends to come back, as not all the fungus cells can be eliminated. Therefore it is expedient to regenerate the bowel flora and strengthen the immune system. This should be done in every case of chronic fatigue syndrome, no matter which agent had been found in that connection.

The cycle of energy production

The role of mitochondria

Having considered all those facts we have come to he conclusion that the state of the immune system plays the most important role in this game. Therefore we have to take a closer look at the factors influencing that system and the terrain on which microbes can thrive, and we will have to find out what leads to conditions that make it harder for them to survive. The energy production, which takes place in our cells, is very important in that context, as that is the main reason for our wellbeing and the proper function of the immune system.

Energy is created in cell organelles, called mitochondria, which are inside the cell body, called cytoplasma. They are the powerhouses of the cell, and their inner membranes are the site of cellular respiration. The energy currency of the body is a substance by the name of ATP (adenosine tri-phosphate), which is created by the electron transport chain in the inner membrane of the mitochondria, in special folds that increase the surface area in the cytoplasma .

In the course of energy production biochemical mediators transport the electrons down that transport chain, where in the end they will react with oxygen. That is the most important way to replenish the body with energy in the form of ATP. This is necessary in every cell of our body, without it no life is possible. All the molecules of the electron transport chain have to flow through the membranes of the mitochondria, so those structures are very important and we should take a closer look at them.

What are cell membranes in general composed of, and what is their function? Cell membranes consist of phospholipid bilayers (double layers) with embedded proteins, they are selectively permeable and the amount of saturated and unsaturated lipids in those layers can differ. The more unsaturated lipids are found in those layers, the more the fluidity of that membrane is increased. Cholesterol, which is also embedded there, confers a stiffening effect to the membrane.

The ratio of phospholipids to cholesterol is different in different cell types, and can even vary in specific cells of the same type. The membranes of the mitochondria are highly permeable for the substances of the electron transport chain and other biochemical substrates such as enzymes. In those mitochondrial membranes the ratio of cholesterol to phospholipids is 0.1. Whereas the ratio in outer cell membranes is 10, as the cholesterol content is much higher there.

This shows the high fluidity of the mitochondrial membranes compared to outer cell membranes. To put it simple, the more cholesterol is laid down in those membranes the less permeable they become, their fluidity then is low.

The role of cholesterol in our metabolism

This leads us to the role of cholesterol in our metabolism, and in order to understand that we have to take a closer look at a few biochemical findings concerning that substance. The name is derived from the Greek word for bile (cholé), as the substance was found in gallstones by a French researcher in 1769.

Cholesterol is a precursor for the biosynthesis of steroid hormones. There are the adrenal gland hormones cortisole and aldosterone, the latter is a mineralo-corticoid, which regulates the levels of sodium and potassium, while it helps to retain sodium. It is part of the renin-angiotensin-aldosterone system, which is important in connection with our blood pressure.

If aldosterone is present in excess, it contributes to the development and progression of cardiovascular and renal disease by influencing blood pressure and distribution of body fluids. It is responsible for the balance of electrolytes in the blood, and stimulates the kidneys to take in more sodium and release potassium. A lack of aldosterone is called Conn's syndrome.

Also the sexual hormones progesterone, the estrogens and testosterone need cholesterol for their production. Furthermore it is essential to produce bile acids and vitamin D. The total body content of Cholesterol is about 35 g, while the daily production is about 1g, and the daily intake of 200-300 mg is depending on the form of nutrition, so that it can be much more or even less than 200 mg.

If our food is rich in cholesterol, this does not automatically mean that our blood cholesterol is raised to high levels. A favourable genetic pattern can prevent that, though a person might eat several eggs per day, which contain plenty of cholesterol.

Besides that the body compensates for absorption of additional cholesterol by reducing the cholesterol synthesis in our own system, genetics seem to play an important role in this context too. Excretion of cholesterol is via bile into the digestive tract, and that can lead to the forming of cholesterol gallstones, if the secretion of bile is sluggish. In that case cholesterol can precipitate in the gall bladder.

Plants on the other hand do not contain cholesterol, but they produce phytosterols instead, substances similar in their chemical structure to cholesterol. And the good message for people who eat plenty of vegetables is, that their phytosterols compete for absorption with cholesterol, and therefore they can lower levels especially of bad cholesterol (LDL); we will discuss this fact later in more detail.

Cholesterol is transported in different forms by using lipoproteins with apolipoproteins acting as ligands (binding sites) directing them to certain tissues. Once bound in tissues it disappears from the blood, and the more binding sites there are in certain tissues, the faster the cholesterol is fixed there, and can do no more harm.

As for lipids there are different transport particles, and it is a rule that the more lipids a particle contains, the less dense it becomes. With increasing density, that means containing more protein, we get the following order: Chylomicrones containing the least protein, very low density lipoproteins(VLDL) are the next, followed by intermediate density lipoproteins (IDL), low density lipoproteins (LDL) and high density lipoproteins (HDL). The last one is the most favourable form, as the cholesterol is bound to protein that prevents unwanted precipitation.

It makes a great difference if the cholesterol is found in the form of High Density Lipoproteins (HDL) or as Low Density Lipoproteins (LDL), as the latter seem to be responsible for the deposition in atherosclerotic plaques in our arteries. The proportion of the two components is dependant on our nutrition, the more fatty acids of the saturated type we eat, the higher the unfavourable LDL cholesterol will be.

To understand the connection we have to consider what (saturated) animal fat is composed of, compared with most vegetable oils, because they are completely different. The main contents of animal fats are triglycerides, consisting of saturated fatty acids and glycerol, then there is cholesterol, and to a lesser extent phospholipids. Elevated triglycerides are an independent risk factor and should also be monitored apart from cholesterol.

Vegetable oils on the other hand contain more unsaturated fatty acids and phytosterols instead of cholesterol, so they counteract the deposition of plaques in our blood vessels.

As animal fat contains plenty of saturated fatty acids, which have been shown to lower the favourable HDL levels and increase LDL, it has been recommended to reduce the intake of saturated fats to less than 7% of the daily energy and the cholesterol intake to less than 200 mg per day.

There also exists the problem of the so-called trans fats, which means that the configuration of the molecule has been changed. Those trans fats, which are mostly created by heating unsaturated vegetable oil for frying, have also been found to increase the amount of LDL cholesterol. Potato chips are mostly fried in vegetable oil, and thus trans fats are created, therefore this form of nutrition should be limited.

The unfavourable LDL cholesterol can be reduced with more phytosterols such as beta-sitosterol contained in high quantities in vegetable oils and nuts, as well as in all kinds of fruit and vegetables. But in the latter they occur in lower quantities. Thus the risk of plaque forming in blood vessels can be lowered.

Because of the similar structure as found in cholesterol, the phytosterols can replace it. The relation of LDL to HDL can be changed in a favourable way by eating more fruit and vegetables. This will protect the arteries from being clogged by plaques, which can lead to heart infarction or brain dysfunction as a consequence of plaque building in blood vessels.

More risk factors for the development of atherosclerosis

1.   Homocystein

But there are more substances that can be hazardous for your blood vessels, the first one is homocysteine, which is a homologue of the amino acid cysteine, an essential sulphur containing amino acid. Elevated levels of homocysteine turned out to be a risk factor for cardio-vascular disease, cognitve impairment such as beginning dementia and even an increased fracture rate in bones. Deficiency in folic acid, pyridoxine (vitamin B6) and cobalamine (vitamin B12) leads to elevated levels of homocysteine and should be substituted. But we did not get an advantage by adding synthetic folic acid to the diet, we got better results instead by changing the diet to a regimen containing more fresh green vegetables.

2. Dimethylargenine

The next risk factor we have to deal with is asymmetric dimethylargenine (ADMA)
It is a risk factor for endothelial dysfunction, which precedes coronary artery disease. Elevated levels of ADMA interfere with the synthesis of nitric oxide (NO) in the endothelium (the inner layer of blood vessels). NO is necessary for endogenous vasodilatation, it inhibits inflammation, adhesion of white blood cells to the endothelium and smooth muscle cell proliferation, therefore NO is a powerful anti-atherosclerotic molecule. The inhibition of NO by ADMA makes it a risk factor and even risk predictor for cardiovascular mortality. ADMA levels are increased in cases of diabetes, hypertension, hypercholesterolaemia, chronic heart failure and chronic renal failure.

3. C-reactive protein (CRP)

Another interesting substance is C-reactive protein (CRP), which is a native protein that is produced in the liver. The levels rise in response to inflammation, and measuring CRP is a screen for infectious and inflammatory diseases, but it does not diagnose a specific disease. Nevertheless it is an independent risk factor for atherosclerotic diseases. Though therapy with statins such as atorvastatin (Lipitor®) is recommended for elevated levels of CRP, we saw no benefit for our patients by doing so. On the contrary, with patients who received statin therapy we saw quite a number of incompatibilities, as for instance elevated muscle enzymes often accompanied by pain.

4. Lipoprotein a

The last substance in that row is lipoprotein a (Lpa), this also has been identified as a risk factor for atherosclerosis, which is manifested as coronary heart disease or stroke. The concentration among people can vary in a wide range; individuals of African descent seem to have higher levels. It has been recommended that people with risk factors should be screened for that substance, if there had been incidents such as early coronary heart disease in the family history. The orthodox therapy consists of niacin in addition to a diet containing less cholesterol and saturated fats or even substances such as atorvastatin (Lipitor®). We had good results with niacin and ginkgo biloba extract; but we would not recommend oestrogen replacement therapy, which had been in use for some time. With that therapy breast cancer rates were found elevated, and even strokes appeared more frequently.

Factors counteracting degenerative diseases

The normal western diet does not meet the criteria for healthy nutrition, as it contains too much saturated fat, thus leading to deposition of LDL cholesterol in foam cells, which were found deposited in blood vessels in the form of plaques.

Besides that we have a lack of trace elements and enzymes in our nutrition, and the amount of helpful substances such as anthocyanins, carotenes and other components of plants, which will be presented in the following list, is also insufficient. These are recommendations for substances that can counteract the risk factors we have been describing in the last chapter.

Anthocyanins

Anthocyanins are plant pigments, which belong to a class called flavonoids. They occur in leaves, flowers and fruit such as blueberries, cranberries, raspberries, blackberries black currants, cherries, grapes, tomatoes, red cabbage, blue soybeans and many others. They are powerful antioxidants and have been found to act favourably on infections, diabetes, cancer, aging and neurological diseases. Some tropical fruit contain a huge amount of it, as for instance the açai berry from South America.

The Carotinoids

The carotinoids are a large group of organic pigments found in chloroplasts and chromoplasts of plants, comprising lutein, xanthin, lycopene and others. They cannot be manufactured in animals and act as antioxidants in various tissues. Carotene has vitamin A activity, as it is a pro-vitamin, and it is necessary for the retina of the eye.

Lutein, an essential corotinoid, protects the retina from blue light, and is recommended for the prevention of macula degeneration. But synthetic supplements of carotenes did not turn out to be beneficial, especially when given to smokers, they seemed to be even hazardous, as cancer rates increased with that regimen.

Huperzine A

The substance called huperzine A is a naturally occurring alkaloid found in the fir moss Huperzia serrata, it is an inhibitor of the enzyme acetyl-cholinesterase. This keeps the enzyme from destroying acetylcholine, which is effective at nerve synapses connecting nerve cells with each other. Therefore huperzine A can improve cognitive performance and enhance memory. The mechanism of action is similar to donepezil (Aricept®), galantamin (Reminyl®) and rivastigmin (Exelon®), which are synthetic substances currently on the market for that purpose. They are supposed to act against neural degeneration as in vascular dementia or Alzheimer's disease. Huperzine A can be bought as a dietary supplement via Internet.

The Salvestrols

The salvestrols are phytoalexins, the word is derived from Greek, alexein meaning to ward off. Plants produce them in response to being attacked by pathogenic organisms such as fungi. The salvestrols are contained in numerous plants and have a slightly bitter taste. There are different classes of salvestrols, they are called alpha, beta, delta and omega salvestrols, the latter seem to be the most effective, they are contained in cabbage and other vegetables and citrus fruit.

In connection with the enzyme CYP1B1, which is present in abundance in cancer cells, they have been found to produce substances, which can attack cancer cells.

Resveratrol belongs to the weaker alpha group, it is contained in fruit such as red grapes and tangerine peel.

The whole resveratrol group seems to be beneficial for cardio-vascular diseases and even diabetes. In animals they have been found to prolong their lifespan and counteract the development of cancer.

Modified citrus pectin (MCP)

Pectin is a carbohydrate made out of numerous polysaccharide molecules, the substance MCP is mostly contained in apples, citrus fruit, especially grapefruit and in plums. In citrus fruit there are altered forms, where the long chain is broken down into smaller soluble fibre molecules, so that it can be absorbed. MCP has been found to help reduce prostate, colon, breast, liver and skin cancer.

S adenosyl methionine (S-AME)

This substance is made out of adenosin-triphosphate (ATP) and the amino acid methionine. It is produced and consumed in the liver, and it is involved in methyl-group transfer, which is important for the metabolism of joints. It was found to reduce pain associated with osteoarthritis. The substance can be bought as a dietary supplement.

Unfortunately many people do not realize that their diet is deficient in many ways, and they often find out about the mistakes they have made much too late, when the damage has already been done. The deposition of waste material begins in early youth with faulty nutrition such as fast food. It contains plenty of saturated fat and lots of sugar, wanting in most of the vital elements we have just described. The whole metabolism can be disturbed that way, and that creates problems with energy supply. It often results in bad circulation, and also leads to imbalances in blood sugar levels that can manifest as diabetes.

The dangers of glycation

When the sugar metabolism is impaired the vicious cycle gets even worse by rigidifying membranes in a process called glycation. This means glucose is attached to cell membranes of red blood cells or to collagen in blood vessels stiffening them, which may lead to the forming of aneurisms. Substantial damage can also be done to structures of the eye such as the lens, cornea and retina, as well as to the beta cells of the pancreas.

The phenomenon of glycation happens on a large scale in diabetic patients whose blood sugar levels have been elevated for a longer period of time, and it can be used for their monitoring by determining the percentage of glycated haemoglobin, as it is proportionate to the length of time.

The transport of oxygen will be impeded by the stiffened membranes, thus leading to problems with energy production and the nutrition of tissues.

In order to change that, the overload of sugar and simple carbohydrates such as white meal products in our nutrition should be changed in favour of complex carbohydrates like wholemeal bread and vegetables. Complex carbohydrates are not digested and transformed into sugar so rapidly, the blood sugar profile can thus be improved. We will discuss nutritional recommendations concerning diabetes later in more detail, as well as plants that can help to get blood sugar levels down.

Influence of radioactivity on our immune system

- Thorium,
- Iodine,
- Caesium,
- Strontium

Thorium

Now we have to compile the facts on substances acting on the immune system and the wellbeing of the whole organism in a noxious way and find out how to counteract those influences. The first example that has been well documented over many years is radioactivity, and so it may serve as a starting point. We will begin the discussion with the formerly widely used contrast agent Thorotrast® containing radioactive Thorium. This substance emits alpha particles, which consist of two protons and two neutrons and are identical to a helium nucleus. This highly ionizing form of particle radiation has a low penetration depth and only becomes dangerous when ingested. Then it can cause various sorts of cancer and leukaemia, as in the case of this contrast agent. It was introduced in 1931, and as it yielded excellent images it was used for more than a decade.

The radioactive particles were stored for a long time in the liver, kidneys, spleen and lymphatic tissue, and led to various kinds of cancer in those organs. It destroyed the immune-active lymphocytes there, and enhanced mutations that turned out to be malignant in nature.

It mostly took more than ten, sometimes more than twenty years, from the injection of the substance to the manifestation of the tumour. So it became clear that the latent period between the incorporation of the toxic substance and the appearance of a tumour is quite long, up to one third of the individual's lifetime.

Thorotrast® was finally abandoned in the 1950's because of the severe long-time effects, but we could learn a lot by closely investigating the whole story of its application.

From the nuclear tests in the 1960's up to the 1990's we know how detrimental radiation can act on the body of humans and animals alike.

A great number of American soldiers, being forced to watch the nuclear testings in the Nevada desert, ended up with all kinds of malignant tumours, and the pictures of the Soviet testings in the Kazakhstan steppe showing mutilated animals are terrible to remember. The British nuclear testings in Southern and Western Australia were of similar outcome, but you did not hear much about the facts for a long time.

Because of considerable latent periods many cancer patients being former soldiers never got recompense for their illness caused by reckless politicians, and that held true for all those above mentioned countries.

Iodine 131

The greatest disaster for Europe was Chernobyl in 1986, and for Asia it was the cataclysmic outcome of the Japanese earthquake and consequent Tsunami on the nuclear reactors of Fukushima in 2011. The Chernobyl disaster was well documented because all of Europe was contaminated by the fallout products, but the worst catastrophe took place in Belorus. The capital of that country, Minsk, is situated in the direction of the wind that blew on the 26th of April in 1986. The first portion hit Minsk heavily bringing a great quantity of radioactive iodine to the city. In the course of several years more and more inhabitants of that region developed carcinomas of the thyroid gland through radioactive iodine. This substance has a relatively short half -life time, namely 8 days, so that it disappeared soon out of the environment.

But more substances had come out of that Ukrainian nuclear reactor that should still be considered.

Caesium

Some other elements stayed in the environment much longer. One of them, radioactive Caesium 137 possesses a half-life of about 30 years, it is a by-product of nuclear fission of Uranium 235.

During nuclear weapon tests and disasters like Chernobyl or Fukushima great quantities of that element were set free. Caesium 137 emits gamma rays, and as it is situated close to potassium in the first row of the periodic system of elements, it is distributed all over the body similar to potassium.

After the Fukushima catastrophe large quantities of Caesium have been found in fish and even in beef. Ingestion of high quantities of radioactive Caesium can be treated with Prussian blue, that way the half-life time is reduced to 30 days, as it is bound chemically.

Caesium 137 can still be found in animals and mushrooms from contaminated areas of Europe, though Chernobyl happened more than 25 years ago.

Strontium

Another element is set free in the course of nuclear fission of Uranium 235, and that is the treacherous Strontium 90. It has an affinity to bones and teeth and stays there for a long time being bound instead of Calcium. The half-life time is more than 18 years, and it belongs into the second group in the periodic system of elements like Calcium. Therefore we understand why it could be found in large quantities in the teeth of children, born shortly after the above ground nuclear testings in the 1950's and 60's.

Those findings were so convincing that President Kennedy signed the Partial Nuclear Test Ban Treaty together with Britain and the Soviet Union in 1961, banning further above ground tests.

Though the nuclear fallout into the atmosphere was decreased after that, we all know that the nuclear testing worldwide went on, using underwater or below ground testing instead. This applied especially to the French tests in the south pacific in French Polynesia, which went on far into the 1990's causing vigorous waves of protest all over the world.

As strontium is mostly accumulated in bones and bone marrow, it could cause bone cancer or leukaemia in people who had been exposed to large doses of radioactivity. This happened to the so-called liquidators who tried to clean up after the Chernobyl disaster and mostly payed with their lives.

We will have to deal with the possibilities of protection against the constant dangers from radioactive contamination later when we talk about other factors of pollution, and what can be done about that.

Consequences of toxic environment and faulty behaviour

One problem with radioactivity lies in the fact that no dose is absolutely harmless, only the probability of detrimental consequences gets higher the higher the dose of radioactivity. Because of the long half-life of several elements there are cumulative effects occurring in the course of time, and in case of a resulting illness such as carcinoma, it will be difficult to find evidence for the connection between the harmful agent and the resulting disease.

So the problem for patients is to prove what substance caused their illness, because much time can have elapsed between the intake of toxins and the manifestation of cancer.

As long as there is no apparent disease, patients do not qualify for any treatment, and once a severe impairment becomes visible it may be too late for efficient treatment.

Some types of cancer like the pancreatic carcinoma are only manifested when they have come into a critical stage, and that considerably diminishes the chances for cure.

Mostly people are left to their own devices to maintain their health and prevent disease with prudent behaviour, and this takes a lot of knowledge, which they have to acquire on their own.

Our approach will be from the standpoint of biological medicine, which is based on the principle of support for the inherent powers of restoration for the body.

Our primary goal will be to correct the underlying causes of disease and to counteract them, so the body can enter into the healing process.

We do not want to replace conventional approaches to treatment of disease, but to add complementary and supportive measures, aimed at improving healing.

It can well be that a patient just wants prophylactic assistance in his efforts to regain or maintain his health.

In the course of this book we will show how the author's experience of over 30 years can contribute to this goal, as the author has worked in all the fields of medicine mentioned here. Orthodox medicine might have been of different opinion concerning therapy in a number of cases, but in consensus with patients we found alternatives and had good results.

The rapid development of the chemical and physical sciences in the past 150 years has had quite an impact on medical thinking and in the course of this development many natural approaches have been forgotten or abandoned, because supposedly better treatment became available with synthetic medication.

But it becomes more and more evident that for instance the treatment of cancer has not shown the kind of progress most scientists had hoped for. It does not appear to be opportune to wait for the miracle drug that will solve our problems with the increasing rate of tumours and many other diseases caused by stress and pollution.

Quite a number of patients are aware of the situation that progress in fighting cancer and chronic diseases has not been rapid in those past decades. All the new and expensive regimens of chemotherapy offered nowadays for cancer treatment in most cases can only postpone the end for a few weeks and at the cost of great suffering. The problem is that we can never reach all the cancer cells by our medication, as they are only vulnerable when in a state of mitosis. But there are always cells, which are not in mitosis, but resting, and so they will not take up the chemotherapeutical substance.

That is why more and more people are looking for an adjunct to their classical therapies, or a way to strengthen their immune system for the prophylactic efforts to maintain their health.

Next we will have to deal with health-destroying living habits or resistance weakened by toxic substances, which are so ubiquitous in our environment.

Faulty nutritional patterns and sluggish metabolism with consequent retention of toxic material together with deficiencies of minerals and trace elements can be considered a major cause of illness together with lack of vitamins and enzymatic cofactors.

Exogenous toxins from polluted air, water and nutrition, tobacco, alcohol and possible intake of drugs create a dangerous cocktail, being even augmented by lack of exercise and emotional stress. Thus we get a health-destroying environment with consequent imbalance in our metabolism, weakening of our detoxifying organs, liver and kidneys, and ineffective assimilation of nutrients.

Considering all those facts it makes more sense to eliminate the causes of disease than to hope for a miracle drug that might take away the self-inflicted condition. By violating the elementary laws of health we compel our body to react with defensive mechanisms such as diarrhoea, pain, fever or complete fatigue.

All those manifestations have the aim to restore a healthy steady state and should not be viewed as the culprit that has to be done away with.

When our body reacts to a virus infection with fever we should not suppress the fever that helps the immune system to get rid of the causative agent. Likewise we should not try to stop diarrhoea indiscriminately, because this can be the way our organism is trying to get rid of toxins or viruses that have caused the irritation.

By interfering with the body's efforts to create its own healing conditions, we often counteract our restoring activity and may well change a condition from acute to chronic, because we do not allow the normal healing process to take place, but try to shorten it.

That means for instance to take antibiotics though the underlying virus infection does not respond to that form of medication. When you feel sick and feverish, it might feel better to suppress the fever and then go to work, but that can result in lasting damage to our body.

With such a behaviour you might trigger the onset of an autoimmune disease, high blood pressure, hardening of arteries, skin eruptions, deposition of toxic waste in joints and connective tissue or even in the lens of the eye, called cataract. Sometimes we also get problems with the vitreous body of the eye, in that case you have the impression that mosquitoes or flies are constantly in your view, because toxic waste is being deposited in that part of the eye in front of the retina.

General considerations on autoimmune processes

Of special interest are the inflammatory diseases in connection with allergies and the immune system.

In the past three decades we have seen an amazing increase of allergies and autoimmune diseases. These auto-aggressive processes are characterised by an attack of immune cells against their own structures, as the immune system in that case seems to consider its own tissues an enemy.

That can literally take place in every part of the body such as the thyroid gland, the kidneys, the liver or the connective tissue and even the nervous system, as in multiple sclerosis.

All those organs can become the target of an autoimmune attack, mediated by our own immune cells called T-lymphocytes.

Normally the activities of those defence cells should be directed against fungi, bacteria, viruses or cells with aberrations as in precancerosis before a cancer becomes manifest. The activities of our immune cells are meant as a protection of the body against everything that is recognised as non-self.

As a matter of fact that can also lead to attacking and rejecting transplanted organs, as they also are non-self.

In those cases the immune system, which tries to reject the foreign organ, has to be suppressed by synthetic drugs to grant the survival of the transplant. But sometimes, when this is not successful, a transplanted organ is nevertheless rejected.

But suppressing the immune system also leads to the consequence that the defence mechanisms against bacteria, viruses and fungi are weakened, and patients in that situation are constantly in danger of falling prey to an infection such as pneumonia.

Virus infections mostly enter our body via the air passages, which can even play an important role in our next complex, as also a large number of allergens are airborne.

General considerations on allergies

First we have to find out what allergy means, as people with ailments in that context have appeared in increased numbers during the past thirty years.

The word was created by the Viennese physician Clemens von Pirquet in 1906 with two Greek words allos and ergon, meaning different work.

Allergies are characterized by antigen-antibody reactions, which cause many problems. Antigens, also called allergens are substances, which under normal circumstances should do no harm, as they mostly are a substance out of the normal environment, which other individuals do not react to.

There are people who are allergic to pollen, animals' hair, dust mites or food ingredients.

Consequences can also appear by reactions to bacterial or virus antigens, which have invaded the body as an infection. As a reaction antibodies are produced, which are proteins called immune globulins, they originate in B-lymphocytes.

A certain type, called IG_E antibodies, can cause an inflammatory response by activating mast cells and basophile white blood cells, which in turn set free allergen mediators such as histamine and leukotrienes.

They can cause hay fever, eczema or asthma, as well as life threatening severe reactions such as anaphylactic shock. Diseases related to allergens such as eczema or asthma have become quite frequent in children, and they are mostly in connection with all kinds of airborne allergens.

Asthma usually gets worse when the child has acquired a respiratory virus, and the virus toxins, acting as allergens, lead to a vicious cycle of spasmodic coughing and the application of synthetic medication to keep the asthmatic symptoms at bay.

The organism reacts by building more cortisole than usual in the adrenal cortex to be able to alleviate allergic symptoms. Thus the immune system is weakened, as the cortisole interferes with the immune functions of lymphocytes, which are important for the defence against viruses and bacteria.

For the recognition of cells that have undergone mutations and should be eliminated special T-lymphocytes are necessary, but cortisole impedes their production and their function.

The orthodox allergy treatment may add even more cortisole besides beta-2 agonists such as salbutamol, antihistamines, adrenaline, theophyllin, cromolyn sodium or anti leukotriens such as montelucast (Singulair®) as a therapy.

The therapy for asthma or eczema could also be tried with homeopathy or Chinese medicine, and in our experience both methods turned out to be quite useful.

Therefore we tried a combination of both, and were surprised to find that we could get even better results by doing so. More details about both ways of treatment will have to be discussed later.

As the roots of those diseases can also be in connection with all kinds of toxins, we will have to speak about those substances first.

Ways of cleansing the body by eliminating foci or toxic tooth fillings

Most conditions of ill health are systemic in their origin, that means not confined to one organ or tissue. So the cleansing of the whole system can be a relief for more than one ailment.

Therefore we will choose the total approach, which means supporting the body's own healing system by cleansing as many organs as possible such as liver, kidneys and connective tissue, at the same time or consecutively and as thoroughly as possible.

That can demand the elimination of toxic amalgams or other materials from tooth fillings, which turned out to be incompatible for that individual. Sometimes certain metals in different teeth are not well tolerated by patients, as a charge can exist between them, and even the plastic material for a prosthetic replacement can cause problems.

Root treatment of teeth can as well lead to chronic foci in the mandible or maxilla of the jaw when decaying tissue is left in the root canal.

Chronically inflamed tonsils with possible pus or scar tissue can be very irritating and cause inflammation in joints, connective tissue, and even the valves of the heart.

Furthermore it should become a rule not to suppress fever reactions, but to give the organism all the rest it needs to cope with an aggressive virus or bacterium if that has invaded the body and led to flu-like symptoms.

Regaining health by proper Nutrition

Doubtlessly one of the most important factors to maintain or restore our health is proper nutrition. How can you be in perfect health if you live for long periods of your life on processed food that had been prepared to be ready in a few minutes in the microwave oven.

Our food should be as fresh as possible, preferably organically grown and only cooked for a short time, not to become some soft mush. It should be, as the Italians say, al dente, so that you can still feel the structure of the ingredients. A substantial portion of our food should be eaten raw; fruit especially loses a lot of its quality when undergoing some sort of cooking or preserving process.

Many vegetables can be eaten as fresh salad, so that there is no need to cook all the available fresh food.

Homemade juices are also well recommended, especially the green drink in the morning out of zucchini, cucumbers, lettuce and onions or garlic.

Juice out of red beets and carrots together with celery and even one raw potato or some cabbage is highly alkaline and helps with ailments like stomach pain, which goes along with reflux of acid into the oesophagus. All sorts of juices are very helpful cleansers, especially when people are on a fast, which should not be undertaken as simple water fasting.

Fasting on the whole can help to lessen ailments caused by type 2 diabetes, which will be discussed in a special chapter. It can also help to cope with the problems of the so called metabolic syndrome, which means high cholesterol, elevated triglycerides and uric acid as well as high blood sugar, frequently accompanied by overweight or even obesity.

It is evident that a lot of our health problems are self-inflicted, and we should not be amazed when we learn that within the past 30 years the percentage of diabetics in western populations has gone up from 3% to now almost 10%.

More food rich in calories is readily available for almost everyone in our countries, and people have to do less and less calorie-burning work, as this can be accomplished by machines. So there is a large discrepancy between the intake of food and the burning of calories by physical work, resulting in the phenomenon of metabolic disturbances caused by obesity.

There is even a strong correlation between the socio-economic status and bodyweight, which is higher with lower socio-economic status of the individual.

This inverse correlation leads to the fact that the life expectancy of poorer people is less because of a higher rate of self inflicted diseases, and not only because the rich get better medical treatment. The key to higher life expectancy lies mostly in the individuals' own behaviour.

General considerations on environmental conditions

This chapter will deal with our environment and what possibilities we have to counteract substances which are hazardous.

Disease producing toxins in air, water, soil and food have caused lots of problems and many companies in the course of aiming at higher profits from their industries have often neglected the fact that they heavily pollute the environment. The threat that better protection of the environment will cost lots of jobs, because it is too expensive, can be used as a pretext to leave everything as it is, thus destroying more and more of the natural resources of our planet.

It is frightening to see how the rainforests in Indonesia and Brazil have dwindled in the last 30 years and how the pollution of rivers for instance in China has killed fish and other living creatures, and made it ever more difficult to supply the people who live in that region with drinking water of an acceptable quality.

We are well aware of the fact that destruction of rain forest is an especially important factor in climate change, and it is not acceptable to grow palm oil plantations in its place, to be able to manufacture so called bio-fuel.

Corn and other grain should not be used for that purpose either, as poorer countries are bereft of their basic nutrients, when the prices for corn or grain rise as a consequence.

From all those facts we can see that saving our planet for future generations does not seem to be the priority for those who can make a profit by their reckless behaviour.

All the mentioned factors are beyond the influence of normal people, unless we can do something by voting for the right government, but that turns out to be illusionary, as no government, regardless of what party, has done enough to protect the environment.

We now turn our attention to the facts that concern people personally and have to be handled as their own responsibility. That means everyone has to think about what poisons may be stored within his or her body, and what can be done do to cleanse them out in order to restore the balance of health.

Let us return to the problems with radioactive substances like iodine 131 that is set free in the beginning of most nuclear disasters.

As our thyroid glands need iodine to produce the hormone Thyroxin, it is essential that nutrition contain that substance. But many people live in a state of chronic deficiency, and so this depleted organ avidly takes up any iodine it can get, even the radioactive variety, as was the case after the Chernobyl disaster. Therefore it is essential to have a good source of iodine to prevent this deficiency and in cases of emergency it is even recommended to take high doses of iodine so the radioactive substance will not be taken up. Only people with latent hyperthyroidism have to be careful, as they may slip into a state of thyrotoxicosis, a severe state of hyperthyroidism with sweating and tachycardia that can become life threatening.

Sodium alginate which is extracted mostly from the brown alga kelp can be helpful, as it is a good chelator, that means capable of a special chemical form of binding, so that it can bind and remove radioactive substances like iodine 131 or

Strontium 90 from our bodies. As not everybody can take a lot of kelp without getting in a state of overactive thyroid gland because of the iodine content, alginate in a purified form without iodine can help to eliminate radioactive substances. It is also advisable to take large amounts of minerals like calcium and magnesium to get a faster turnover of radioactive elements such as strontium 90.

Toxic Heavy metals

Let us next look at the toxic metals cadmium, lead and mercury, which have been present in our environment for several generations and still can cause major health problems, as not enough has been done to replace them in our immediate environment.

Cadmium

Cadmium is known to afflict our body in a detrimental way The kidneys and arteries are especially vulnerable to cadmium, as it can cause atherosclerosis with high blood pressure, heart problems and many more.
The sources of cadmium are manifold from air, polluted by auto exhaust fumes, to all kinds of goods contaminated by cadmium. Examples of these can be toys from China or even mushrooms, which have grown not far from polluting industries, as they tend to concentrate cadmium out of the air. Tap water can contain it because of the manufacturing of the piping, and it does not seem to be safe to drink tap water unless it has been proven that in your environment cadmium actually is not present in larger amounts.

So what can be done to get protection from the detrimental influence of cadmium? It is important to know that the trace element zinc is an antagonist to cadmium, as a consequence foods rich in zinc like whole meal products or nuts should be consumed in abundance or the element should be given as a supplement.

Enamelled products such as bowls for salads should be avoided, because the acid tends to dissolve cadmium from the enamel, and in times of cheap import products the danger is still present though the problem has been known for several decades.

Livers and kidneys of animals concentrate cadmium and it is advisable to abstain from these as well as from tap water if heavy metals can be found in it.

Lead

The next element we want to take a closer look at is lead.

Dating back to the time when lead was used worldwide as tetra-ethyl lead as an additive to automobile fuels we still have lead contamination in the environment.

There are other sources, which add to that load, for example, lead containing paint, ceramic glazes, industrial production or recycling of lead batteries.

Nevertheless lead contamination has significantly decreased since it has been banned as an additive to automobile fuels. But unfortunately it has not been abandoned in kerosene for aeroplanes.

So with heavy air traffic lead is coming down through the air, and people inadvertently take up this dangerous substance.

It is especially hazardous for children, because it interferes with brain development and can lead to behavioural and learning disorders.

Lead is also toxic for the blood building organs, as it impairs the haemoglobin synthesis.

It is also hazardous for the nervous system, as it interferes with the action of neurotransmitters, which are used by neurons to send out signals to other cells.

On top of that lead enhances cell death in brain cells.

It can also affect the intestines, the kidneys, the heart and the reproductive system.

Thus lead can lead to anaemia, seizures and coma or produce insomnia, delirium, cognitive deficits, tremor or abdominal pain.

By taking the place of calcium, iron or zinc in certain enzymes it can interfere with the action of those enzymes and make them inefficient.

Though all this has been known for a long time, there are still many houses where lead paint or lead piping are in use, thus releasing that element into the air or into tap water.

As it is also nephro-toxic, it can lead to kidney damage, elevated blood pressure, coronary heart disease, stroke and cataract formation, (meaning waste material is deposited in the lens of the eye.)

Blood and urine tests can show lead poisoning, making it necessary in severe cases not only to avoid further exposure, but also to eliminate the substance. We will later show how this can be done with chelating agents.

Besides that it makes sense to substitute calcium, iron and zinc and to add lecithin to the nutrition to protect the brain.

Homeopathic treatment can enhance the excretion by using plumbum sulphuricum in a higher potency such as C30. The homeopathic substance will help to lead out the toxic element, (plumbum is the Latin word for lead).

In Chinese medicine there are also formulas that help to detoxify poisonous substances, and it is always important to strengthen the organs, which are occupied with that task such as liver and kidneys. A list of Chinese herbs and formulas will follow in another chapter at the end of this book.

Mercury

Next thing the problem of Mercury poisoning has to be dealt with, as that element can cause kidney, lung and brain damage with sensory impairment, disturbed sensation and lack of coordination, as well as peripheral neuropathy and paraesthesias, (which means feeling disorders).
Especially dangerous are organic mercury compounds, which can be ingested with sushi or other dishes from big fish.
These fish are higher on the food chain, and they have already concentrated toxic substances by devouring other creatures lower on the food chain. Tuna and whale meat for that reason contain plenty of mercury, though the whale is not a fish.
Mercury inhibits selenium dependant enzymes, which can lead to inability to degrade the catecholamines adrenaline and noradrenaline, resulting in symptoms such as sweating, hypertension, tachycardia or insomnia. Kidney dysfunction, mental lability and memory impairment can also result from toxic mercury, as well as desquamation of the skin.

Mercury toxins can be found in fish, florescent lamps, which are advertised as energy savers and amalgam fillings of teeth. Coal plants, crematoria and gold production can also be the source of this heavy metal.

Another problem is a preservative called Thiomersal, an organic mercury-containing substance used in vaccines, which can lead to reactions in patients. Fortunately, with the exception of influenza vaccines, most vaccines are nowadays free of that substance.
Liquid mercury on the other hand is poorly absorbed, so that people who by accident ingest the contents of a broken thermometer mostly survive without any major impairment. Mercury vapour that can be absorbed through the respiratory tract or methyl mercury, which can even penetrate the skin, are much more dangerous.
As those mercury compounds can be created in the body of people having amalgam fillings, there are several countries like Norway, which have banned amalgam from use in dentistry, because it could no longer be considered as safe.

Chelating agents to remove toxic heavy metals

For cleansing procedures of heavy metal residues there exists a new chelating agent. This was developed by the Russian military and can eliminate toxic heavy metals from our body. It is available under the name DMPS or Dimaval®, the exact name is 2,3 Bi-sulfonyl-propane-1-sulfonic acid.
We have a very active chelating substance containing sulphur that can grab heavy metals in tissues of the body and lead them out via kidney excretion.

A chelate is a complex chemical compound, by which metals can be bound and led out. A similar substance is DMSA that acts in a similar way to DMPS, available not only in ampoules, but also in capsules; sometimes patients tolerate this better than the DMPS. In our opinion those two substances are superior to EDTA or DMSO, which can be used for similar purposes to get rid of toxic heavy metals.

The author of this book has worked with the first two substances for a number of years and has never seen any serious side effects if handled with care and responsibility, having had quite rewarding results in cases of mercury and lead poisoning.

Dimaval® may be difficult to obtain in some countries, as Medical Associations put restrictions on its use.
The acting of Dimaval® is rapid, and we can detect a rise to the hundredfold of toxic metals in the urine within two hours after injection, compared to the urine before the injection. Nevertheless it is only recommended for severe cases, otherwise it is expedient to use DMSA capsules.

It makes sense to simultaneously substitute important trace elements like Zinc, Manganese, Selenium or the macro element Magnesium.
In the course of eliminating toxic heavy metals we can create losses of trace elements and minerals in general, so also Calcium and other minerals should be substituted to make up for these losses.
By supporting the liver and kidneys with Chinese herbs, as will be explained more thoroughly later, we help these organs to cleanse out their toxic residues. The author has

never seen any patient who had been treated with that therapy suffer or not feel well, if enough support was given to the excreting organs.

In severe cases of heavy metal intoxication we usually deal with this problem by using chelating agents such as DMPS or DMSA to lead out the toxic elements via kidney elimination.

In less severe cases we can use another interesting substance to get rid of mercury and other heavy metals by giving patients Chlorella algae, pressed in tablets. They bind toxic metals to its surface and lead them out via bowel elimination without causing any side effects.
It goes without saying that before we start to detoxify, amalgam fillings should be removed from teeth, in order to avoid permanent new mercury poisoning out of these fillings.

Here again mineral supplements are recommended, as well as lecithin because of the neurotoxicity of mercury.
The central as well as the peripheral nervous system can be affected by mercury and other heavy metals, and it can also lead to psychological or psychiatric problems such as depression.

Problems related to platinum and worldwide traffic

Since tetraethyl lead has been banned as an additive in car fuels, we created another problem by using platinum for catalytic converters in automobiles.

It remains questionable if this is a good solution, since platinum can form dangerous radicals and other toxic components, which are suspected of causing alveolar lung cancer.

As yet this problem has not been given due attention.

So how can the problem of auto traffic becoming more every year worldwide be solved?

Maybe the electro-car or the hydrogen driven engine can diminish the problems with pollution. In both cases we are confronted with problems, because the current to charge up car batteries, will have to be obtained by mostly burning fossil energy carriers like coal, oil or gas, thus adding to the worldwide CO_2 production.

This is said to cause climate change, as the percentage of power from other sources such as sun, wind and water is not very high in most countries

With hydrogen we have a different problem, because it cannot easily be stored, and it is an explosive.

The aforementioned bio fuels have to be seen critically, because they are made out of palm oil or grain and deprive the world's population of their urgently needed food sources.

Using tidal energy is as yet a future project, as well as the research on free energy.

So probably cars driven by solar energy will be the most promising attempt to get away from fossil energy carriers. We will be able to save on oil by using solar panels as an adjunct to the Diesel or petrol engine in the near future.

A few car manufacturers already offer this combination.

That way CO_2 output could be decreased and air quality in cities would become better.

Smog from auto fumes contains hundreds of toxic components besides carbon monoxide, nitrogen dioxides and many other substances. Carbon monoxide output is dangerous, as it deprives the cells of oxygen, and therefore great efforts were made to diminish it by using platinum catalysts.

But this advantage had to be bought at a high price, because platinum is not as innocuous as one would wish. It was found that the rates of alveolar lung cancer skyrocketed in California a few years after the introduction of catalytic converters in that state in the 1970's, probably because of the carcinogenous potential of that metal.

For most of the exhaust toxins there is no specific way of elimination.

German doctors Voll and Hagen created a system of detoxification by homeopathy, but most people never heard of that.

Therefore the most important way of prophylaxis consists of avoiding an overload of these components and getting plenty of oxygen by doing exercise in clean air.

Breathing and exercises

When it comes to proper breathing it is amazing to see how many people seem to be unaware of their respiration being too shallow. A great number of women turn out to be unable to use deep respiration by lowering their diaphragm, when they are told to breathe into their abdomen in order to get more space for their lungs.

So a good exercise for that purpose can be to lie on your back and place a book on your abdomen. When you inhale the book should come up, because the diaphragm is being lowered pushing the abdomen out. As you exhale the book is coming down, as the diaphragm is moving upward bringing the abdomen back into the original position.

By relaxing and breathing slowly and deeply, more oxygen is taken up, and in the long run even the vital capacity of the lungs will be extended.

That will consecutively lead to more oxygen in all the cells, and thus the electron transport chain can be enhanced creating more ATP, our energy currency, as was explained in the chapter on mitochondria.

Proper breathing has to be learned first and then a program of physical exercises can be outlined for individual use. Exercise is very important for the wellbeing of everyone, as the muscle pump helps a great deal with the transport of the venous and lymph system, which is important for detoxifying the body. This will lead to sweating, which is a good way to get rid of toxic substances that should not be underestimated. It is expedient to slowly build up a program for individual use, in order not to demand too much in the beginning, especially for people who already have joint or heart problems. Otherwise you may do more harm than good for your body. All the structures of muscles, ligaments and tendons must gradually be adapted to a workout or jogging regimen. Then it will be an invaluable means to get more oxygen into the system by better breathing, training your circulation, and even the perfusion of vital organs such as the heart muscle will be improved.

People who already have some trouble with the cartilage in their joints, should go swimming or ride a bicycle, which for them is better than jogging, because it does not put all the weight on these joints.

For young people jogging can be recommended, but it does not make sense to do so on a street with heavy traffic, as the auto fumes contain lots of toxins and free radicals that react with cell membranes. Thus our energy metabolism can be impaired or even DNA mutations can occur, which could be the reason for later development of cancer. Antioxidants are needed to help the body to get rid of these hazards of civilisation.

Antioxidants and nutritional balance

Because of the heavy load of free radicals in our environment plenty of antioxidants are essential, as we all cannot evade the risks of civilisation completely. These substances are natural vitamin E, Vitamin C, beta- carotene, anthocyanins and also additional zinc, manganese, chromium, copper and selenium and many others.

They are necessary for the production of detoxifying enzymes such as superoxide dismutase. This enzyme dismutates (transforms) superoxides into oxygen and hydrogen peroxide, and therefore is a defence for all cells.

There are different forms of this enzyme, depending on the location inside or outside of cells.

It can be found in the cytoplasm or in the mitochondria, in the latter case the enzyme is connected to the trace element manganese.

If this enzyme is defective a severe consequence can result, and that is Lou Gehrig's disease, also called Amyotrophic Lateral Sclerosis or Moto-Neuron Disease, which can result in showing weakness, muscular atrophy and fasciculations, that means involuntary twitching of muscles. In the end these patients have problems speaking (dysarthria), swallowing (dysphagia) and breathing (dyspnoea). When a patient gets into such a life-threatening state, assisted respiration will be needed and feeding by a tube.

The aforementioned aggressive free radicals have an unpaired number of electrons and are very reactive, therefore they can destabilise other molecules and become a hazard for numerous body structures such as cell membranes. Even the genetic information in our DNA can be changed by free radicals. We will discuss later how this happens.

Antioxidants are necessary to terminate the chain reactions that have been started by free radicals in order to protect cell membranes.

There are plenty of antioxidants in fresh unprocessed foods, and therefore it makes sense to have the sort of nutrition that contains all these ingredients in combination with vegetable oil containing unsaturated fats to grant a good supply of the essential fatty acids.

Proteins should not be consumed in excess because they can leave toxic end products. Especially excessive protein consumption of animal source like meat has turned out to lead to toxic decomposition in our bowel, and therefore the intake of meat should not be too copious. The hazard of cancer in the large bowel decreases notably if meat intake is restricted.

Apart from that red meat has turned out to be a risk factor in respect to atherosclerosis. It leads to an overload of carnitine, which results in the production of a toxic substance called TMOA (trimethylamine N-oxide).

This substance is associated with atherosclerosis, as the transport of cholesterol is hindered, and it can be deposited in atherosclerotic plaques. This happens mostly in people who consume red meat regularly and have a TMAO producing bowel flora.

This alteration of the bowel flora does not occur with persons who live mostly on vegetarian food and seldom or never eat red meat.

In a normal range carnitine is necessary for the long chain fatty acid transport in our metabolism, therefore it is considered to be an essential substance when the balance is kept and the bowel flora is healthy.

Another important aspect is the amount of grain that is necessary to produce one kilogram of meat, as many farmers in the United States feed their cattle with grain. It can be up to twenty kilogram for a single kilogram of meat.

In view of a growing world population that is threatened by hunger this is not acceptable.

People who are not so dependant on meat can easily go on a meat free nutrition and will profit even more.

All the essential amino acids are contained in vegetable sources that are readily available like nuts, seeds, grains or legumes, preferably in combination, such as the combination of rice and soybeans, as used in Asia, or maize and dried beans being the combination of Central and South America. These sources of protein are complementary and all the essential amino acids are contained therein.

The whole system will profit from the aforementioned nutrition, and it will also help to get rid of toxins, as less meat means less acid forming food.

If there is a lot of acidity in our tissues the deposition of waste material takes place to a larger extent leading to stiffening and swelling of joints and connective tissue.

To counteract all those detrimental consequences it is recommended to eat more food, which is alkaline-forming, that means fruit and vegetables with the addition of trace elements and minerals.

Though some fruit may be sour to taste, it turns out to be alkaline in the course of digestion, as the organic components such as citric acid will be completely metabolised in the Krebs cycle, also called citric acid cycle.

This does not hold true for instance for acetic acid, which is formed by digesting fats. Long chain fatty acids of the saturated type have to be broken down into small acetyl molecules, which have to be burned in the citric acid cycle.

But sometimes the citric acid cycle cannot cope with an overload of those molecules, leading to acidosis in the body with many detrimental consequences such as deposition of waste material in joints and connective tissue.

Besides that impaired absorption of trace elements and minerals like calcium occurs due to acidosis. But minerals such as calcium are necessary not only for our bones, but also for blood clotting and nerve function. Especially in diabetic patients the building of the toxic substance acetone out of sour acetyl molecules is a feared consequence of metabolic imbalance of fatty acids, which goes along with blood sugar problems.

Another substance that has nothing to do with nutrition, but can endanger people having to work with, is our next point.

Problems with asbestos

Asbestos is a set of naturally occurring silicate fibres, which has been known for several thousand years. It was named after a town in the province of Québec, Canada, where the mining on a large scale started in modern times, which now takes place mostly in Russia, China, Brazil and Kazakhstan.

Even in ancient times it was used because of its resistance to fire. During the past 150 years it was sought after as heat and electrical insulation material, for sound absorption and for insulation in buildings, often mixed with cement or woven into mats.

The inhalation of the thin fibrous crystals, which are invisible for our eyes, can cause a number of serious illnesses. The worst ones are the malignant pleura mesothelioma and lung cancer, which occur after long-term exposure to airborne particles. But most people ended up with asbestosis, when they had worked in the mining, as construction workers or auto mechanics. The hazard came from replacing brake pads and shoes, which for decades contained asbestos.

So what does it mean to get asbestosis?

Asbestosis is a sort of fibrosis of the lungs or thickening of the pleura, where asbestos fibres have been caught. This leads to impaired respiration with severe consequences for the whole metabolism.

On the outer skin asbestos warts can develop if asbestos fibres get stuck between skin cells. All this happens through mechanical damage, and in the long run the permanent irritation can lead to inflammation. The development of lung carcinoma or pleura mesothelioma has an incubation time of 12 to 20 years, similar to many other cancers. In most countries this has been recognized as work related disease, and the substance has been banned. But there are more than 200 thousand cases of litigation still pending alone in the United States.

As long as the substance is bound in cement or tiles, not so many fibres are airborne, most dangerous are parts where fibres can be easily set free.

Unfortunately there exists no possibility to get the fibres out once they are stuck in lung or pleura tissue. Therefore exposure should be prevented in any possible way by getting rid of all asbestos containing parts in a house. The treatment of asbestosis can only be symptomatic, with oxygen or antibiotics in case of bronchitis or pneumonia.

As for treatment with Chinese herbs or homeopathy there are remedies for lung and bronchial ailments that can also help to alleviate the symptoms of asbestosis.

The ozone dilemma

As there is some confusion concerning that topic, we want to clarify the action of ozone in different layers around the earth (the atmosphere).

Ozone (O_3) is a pollutant in the troposphere (ground level) where animal life takes place on earth. It is created from the combustion of fossil fuels by the action of ultraviolet light. That means the more traffic we have, the more ozone will be created, especially during the summer month with plenty of UV light.

Ozone can harm lung function and cause asthma, bronchitis or heart attacks, as well as irritation of mucous membranes of eyes and nose. The ozone in the stratosphere, 10-50 km above surface, on the other hand is not a pollutant, instead it acts as protection against excessive ultraviolet light.

During the past decades it has declined because of certain substances called chlorofluorocarbons (CFCs) and similar molecules. They gradually destroyed part of the protective ozone layer of the stratosphere. CFCs were used as frigerants and propellants, that means as cooling agents in refrigerators and in all kinds of sprays for asthma and other use.

In the stratosphere ozone filters out sunlight and UV light, the unabsorbed part of which causes sunburn in humans. It can also damage the DNA in living tissues of humans, animals and plants. As a consequence skin cancer rates were increasing in countries such as Australia with intense sun light. The so-called ozone hole is worse in countries farther away from the equator, as in the Arctic and the Antarctic region and adjacent countries, especially on the southern hemisphere. We should do all we can to keep the protective ozone layer in the stratosphere from further diminishing.

Therapies for irritated mucous membranes from ozone can be similar to allergy therapies with homeopathic remedies.
For eye problems due to ultraviolet light Euphorbia as eye drops can be helpful.
We will give more details when talking about remedies for mucous membranes at the end of this book.

General considerations on fasting

To enhance detoxifying processes, it can be recommended to go on a fast. The flushing out of toxins is accomplished more quickly, and people can recover more easily from all sorts of ailments. A proper fasting regimen should also comprise the cleansing of the bowels with daily enemas. Hydro colonic procedures, which act as more intense enemas twice a week, can help to cleanse the bowel faster and more thoroughly.
Lots of toxins can be eliminated from the bowels that way, and it is amazing to see how well patients feel on a fast, as they are able to undergo physical exertions of all kind.
This could be mountain climbing or going on longer hikes for several hours in a row.

The author of this book has worked in a fasting clinic with thousands of patients for several years and has seen people greatly profit in every possible respect from fasting.
All kinds of positive reactions can occur by fasting, from improvement of blood sugar in diabetics, to lessening of pain in patients with arthritis and better general health.
The purpose of fasting is always to improve health, and the loss of weight is only a by-product of the process. Nevertheless the weight loss itself can bring some important changes.

For instance, in type2 diabetics we see better blood sugar profiles when patients lose some of their overweight.
There have been lots of controversies about fasting during the past decades and what to expect of it, so let us consider the history of fasting first.

Fasting is an ancient therapeutic method, as men and even animals instinctively stop eating when they are not feeling well, until their health is restored. But with modern drug-oriented medicine fasting lost more and more of its attraction.

It was stated by orthodox physicians that a body on a fast would lose too much of its vital proteins by digesting its own muscle mass. Therefore it was demanded that at least some protein should be administered to keep the body structures from shrinking.

In the author's own experience, of being a doctor in a fasting clinic, things like that never happened.

Though we put patients on fasts for up to 6 weeks, without giving them protein substitutes during the fasting period, no negative outcome has ever been seen.
The same experience was published by colleagues in Europe who have run fasting clinics for many decades in Germany, Spain, Switzerland and Sweden.

They all state that fasting is safe, and they never saw side effects like heart muscle loss as a consequence. Nor did they observe weakness due to loss of muscle in the extremities. On the contrary fasting patients felt strong and rejuvenated even after long periods of getting no solid food but just fresh vegetable juice, herbal tea and freshly made vegetable broth without salt.

The importance of the intestinal flora for the whole system

Cleansing the bowel should be considered an important part of the therapy, and as the bowel flora is a highly complex system we should take a closer look at it.

The intestine of a human being contains about 100 trillion microorganisms, that is ten times as much as all our body cells.

Sixty percent of the dry mass of faeces consists of bacteria, and the species Bacterioides normally comprises about 30% of the whole flora. Certain bacteria are essential for our digestive processes, and they can also produce vitamins, such as vitamin K.

They can prevent growth of harmful, pathogenic germs such as Salmonella or an overgrowth with fungi like Candida.

The intestinal flora of a baby is built up during the first few weeks of his or her life by contact with the mother and other persons that come into close contact.

In breast-fed infants a high percentage of Lactobacillus can be found, which seems to be quite favourable, as the intestinal flora helps train our immune system, which can prevent allergies.

Every individual has a somewhat different bowel flora, and it depends on the nutritional habits and other circumstances in this person's life how the flora develops or is changed.

There are many different types of bacteria in our bowel; most of them are anaerobes, that means they live without oxygen.

The largest portion are Bacterioides, and besides that you can find Escherichia coli, Clostridia, Ruminococcus, Bifidobacter, Peptostreptococcus, Lactobacillus acidophilus, and many more.

All the different bacteria in our normal intestinal flora should exist in an appropriate proportion to each other in order to keep the system in a balanced state.

In case of bowel problems, after the intake of antibiotics or chemotherapy, the intestinal flora can be severely damaged. So a careful therapy to build up a new healthy flora is advisable.

Because of the complexity of functions there are also effects on the immune system. It is well known that the immune organ called Peyer's patch is situated beneath the mucous membrane of the small bowel. Those structures are similar to lymphatic nodules. They constitute the immune system of the bowel and are important for the whole organism. Seventy percent of the lymphatic tissue, to be found in the whole organism, is located in the small bowel.

In case of damage to the flora, when the good symbiotic bacteria have been diminished, and Acidophilus and Bifidus bacteria are no longer there in a sufficient quantity, also the Bacteriodes count can be too low.

They are often replaced by overgrowth of unwanted Ruminococcus, which disturbs the whole balance of the flora.

It gets really dangerous if the number of Clostridium difficile becomes too high, as this aggressive germ creates a sort of colitis that is called pseudomembranous, which is accompanied by severe diarrhoea.

This can happen after antibiotics have been taken for a long time and no help was given to build up a new healthy flora.

There are preparations on the market in the form of capsules or liquids, which will help to regenerate the bowel flora after it has been damaged. They are called probiotics, containing live Acidophilus and Bifidus bacteria cultures.

There are also substances available to regenerate a normal flora of Escherichia coli by taking capsules of Mutaflor®. They contain a certain strain of E. coli, isolated in 1917 by Nissle in Germany, which showed good results even in the treatment of ulcerative colitis. We saw more favourable results with that regimen than we saw after the treatment with synthetic remedies for all forms of colitis

Outbreaks of disease occurred from time to time with very aggressive strains of Escherichia Coli, as for instance the EHEC variety, meaning Entero-Hepatic Escherichia Coli.

This strain caused a severe epidemic outbreak in northern Germany in 2011, extending from there over several European countries. It was triggered by contaminated sprouts grown out of seeds from Egypt, which had been distributed over a large area. More than 50 people died of liver and kidney failure in the course of this outbreak, and more than 500 had been severely ill from this inflammation.

So how can an organism cope with lesions of inflammatory nature such as in colitis?

A certain class of proteins has become interesting in connection with bowel inflammations when lesions of the intestinal tract mucosa had appeared.

Those proteins are called Toll Like Receptors (TLR), and they play a role in the innate immune system. They are expressed in immune cells like macrophages, which are a subpopulation of lymphocytes, or in dendritic cells. The latter are immune cells that present antigen material to other cells of the immune system.

TLR can recognise certain molecules from microbes once these microbes have breached the mucosa of the intestinal tract, then as a consequence they activate immune cell responses.

The TLR received their name because of the similarity to the Toll gene, which was identified in the fruit fly Drosophila melanogaster in 1985 by Christiane Nuesslein-Volhard in Germany. This gene plays a role in the fly's immunity to fungal infections by activating the synthesis of antimicrobial peptides.

In humans TLR were described first by Nomura in 1994.

Those molecules seem to be able to repair damage of the bowel walls, which is a very important finding concerning lesions caused by inflammatory diseases of the intestines.

With a healthy flora this repairing process seems to function quite well, but with unfavourable changes in that flora the healing process is slowed down considerably.

From all those facts it becomes evident how important a healthy intestinal flora is for the wellbeing of a person, and that it is difficult to maintain a proper flora, if the entire body chemistry is not in balance.

In that case harmful organisms will easily gain a foothold, because it takes a proper balance of minerals and vitamins, as well as a balance of acids in our metabolism for proper function. Otherwise the internal environment will not support a healthful bowel flora.

The normal western diet does not meet the criteria necessary for healthy nutrition, as it is on the acid side and contains too much meat. This causes an environment of rotting in our intestines, as meat fibres are hard to digest.

There are also too many empty calories in that food consisting of much sugar, white bread and soft drinks and too much fat of the saturated type.

On the whole we have food of poor quality, as it usually contains residues of pesticides and all sorts of additives such as preservatives, colourings, emulsifiers, flavourings and artificial sweeteners like aspartame.

Our drinking water is mostly contaminated with chlorine, fluoride and other chemicals like residues of chemical drugs, which can interact with our whole system, especially the hormones and the intestinal flora.

We do not hold the opinion that fluoride should be added to drinking water, because we had several young patients who had become sick by taking fluoride as tooth prophylaxis against caries for several years. The symptoms promptly disappeared when the intake of those pills was cancelled.

The symptoms had been in a broad range from abdominal cramps to mental problems. We think everybody should have the freedom to decide if he wants to take fluoride, and no one should be forced to take a substance that is potentially harmful, but is constantly present in our drinking water.

Besides that we do know better ways to keep tooth decay at bay by taking care of adequate nutrition and staying away from all that sugary stuff children and adults are coaxed to buy when seeing all those stupid commercials on TV or elsewhere.

It should be a major goal to have water of high quality, as it is the most important substance for our lives, and the replacement especially after sweating is essential.

But we know that many people do not drink enough, as adults need about two litres of water every day, sometimes more, if there had been considerable losses. Otherwise the kidneys will have to do the heavy work of concentrating the urine to a large extent, and may not be able to flush out all the toxins that could harm the body.

So our drinking water should not be contaminated with all sorts of chemicals or residues of pharmaceuticals and agricultural substances such as nitrates out of mineral fertilizers. All those substances not only harm the intestinal flora, but can also become carcinogens.

Antibiotics, especially of the wide spectrum type, often destroy a valuable part of our bowel flora allowing other bacteria, fungi and parasites to grow unimpeded. After a course of antibiotics every physician should recommend a regimen of probiotic bacteria in order to regenerate the intestinal flora.

Other drugs interfere with the digestion of our food, as for instance acid-blockers, painkillers and anti-inflammatory drugs. They have to be detoxified by the liver thus leading to new problems, as the liver is flooded by an overload of work. This organ has to bear the burden of all the toxic heavy metals and residues of insecticides and the like in our nutrition anyway.

Stress and mental tension can also affect the digestive process, leading in some cases to overeating and in others to states of anorexia or bulimia.

Under such pathological conditions we cannot expect to find a healthy flora, instead we can see some of the following symptoms occurring, which are typical for an unbalanced state.

Bloating and excessive gas building are signs of improper digestion. Foul smelling stools show decomposition of proteins, when the ingested quantity was too high, and the proteins cannot be digested properly.

Diarrhoea, cramping or constipation are signs that the whole intestinal system is in a state of severe imbalance.

The same holds true, if weakness, sleepiness or headaches appear after a meal.

We should do everything to restore a favourable intestinal flora and thus keep pathogenic and harmful organisms at bay.

To improve the whole metabolic balance we have to start with cleansing our body structures, thus slowing down the aging process, as the clogging of our detoxifying system interferes with the regeneration of our tissues.

We know that disease begins as a slow process, as the deposition of waste products interferes with oxygenation and nourishment of our cells. With sluggish metabolism and nutritional deficiencies, lack of exercise, overeating and poor digestion our cells start to degenerate, and in the end the whole system will break down resulting in illness or death.

How to clean the body by fasting

Dying cells should be decomposed and eliminated from the body as fast as possible to make room for new regeneration. At this point juice fasting comes in as an effective way to help with the elimination of body waste and speeding up regeneration. On a fast that is longer than a few days, our body will live on its own substance and will start decomposing and digesting its own structures, but not indiscriminately.

It will start with cells that are diseased or damaged, thus feeding on all the material that has become inferior and is no longer fit for a healthy being. It is a kind of waste disposal in a specific way, leaving the essential organs undamaged.

In the course of that procedure even tumours can be destroyed and excreted or digested as we have seen in a number of cases. Toxic waste from organs like liver, kidneys, lungs and bowel is expelled at a faster rate enabling these organs to regenerate.

We can see by checking uric acid levels that usually they become elevated during a fast, because deficient cells are decomposed faster, and more uric acid than normally is thus produced.

When all that waste is coming out it can result in the fasting symptoms of strong smelling sweat, offensive breath, dark urine and discharge of various body fluids.

By fasting assimilative organs get some rest, and after that the utilisation of food and the digestive process is markedly improved. So on the whole we have a stabilizing and rejuvenating effect for the whole body.

That is why we have seen so many favourable changes in general health, as well as in specific situations of rheumatic and metabolic diseases in people undergoing that procedure.

In animals it can be shown that their lifespan is greatly increased by making them fast from time to time, best on a regular basis.

So fasting is not only safe but can be highly recommended for various ailments. The next question is, which is the best way of fasting, and for how long can I go on a fast.

As already mentioned we would not recommend water fasting. By giving patients fresh juices made out of fruit or vegetables and adding herbal tea and vegetable broth we see much better results.

This is understandable as vitamins, minerals, enzymes and trace elements can be found in the aforementioned regimen of fasting, adding alkaline fluids to the body that in a fast tends to form acids in the process of cleansing. The body's healing activity is augmented and sped up and the cell regeneration will take place more easily.

Mineral imbalances can thus be eliminated and when the cell oxygenation is increased it leads to a slowing down of aging processes.

The length of people's fast depends on several different aspects, especially on health issues that have already arisen. Then we should consider the time a patient wants to spend on fasting, and what is expected of it.

Generally spoken people who go on a fast for the first time should try 5 to 10 days of fasting, the more experience they acquire, the longer they will want to fast, because they detect all the beneficiary aspects of it.

We had people fasting from 5 days up to 6 weeks, and all of them held the opinion that they had felt really good during that time.

The initial feeling of hunger diminishes quickly and from the third day on most patients have no hunger at all, feeling light and easy and being in a good mental state.

Before the fasting begins we would recommend to go on a light fruit and raw vegetable diet, with salads made of all available fresh vegetables that can be eaten raw.

On the first day of fasting it can be helpful to start the day with a glass of water containing one teaspoon full of Glauber's salt. That is a hydrated sodium sulphate which was found by the German physician Johann Rudolf Glauber in an Austrian spring in 1625.

This salt will help to cleanse the bowel initially, and then on the following days patients start with their daily enema.

Twice a week they get a hydro-colonic instead, which leads to an even more intense cleansing.

In the morning the fasting patient is given half a litre of herbal tea, and later on one glass of freshly pressed vegetable juice. At noon the lunch consists of half a litre of vegetable broth that has to be cooked for 45 minutes by using lots of fresh vegetables. The cooking time has to be that long to get the rich minerals out of the vegetables. We do not add salt, as most people take too much of that anyway, and it retains water in the tissues.

Herbal tea can be drunk any time as much as anyone wants, and it should be more than one litre per day. In the afternoon fresh fruit juice should be available, especially appreciated on hot days. In the evening again 1 glass of vegetable juice and tea will be given to everyone on a fast.

As the Glauber's salt should be given only on the first day, on consecutive days the fasting patient should apply his daily enema, only to be substituted for a colonic on two days during the first week.

In case of severe bowel problems hydro-colonics can be given for the whole length of the fasting, once or twice a week. That sounds all fairly easy, and in reality does not pose too many problems. Not quite so easy is the time when patients break their fast and have to be put on a careful regimen to be brought back to normal eating.

That has to be done over several days and depends on the length of the fast. The longer an organism has been deprived of food the more time it will take to reacquaint it to normal eating. So on the day of breaking the fast we must not make the mistake to give too much food too soon, and nothing fried or fatty should be eaten. Best thing is to start with a light vegetable soup without any fat or we grate a raw potato into boiling water thus creating a nice potato soup. A little salt may be added, and patients always like this first meal. From then on you have more freedom to choose your food, but it still should be light and not too copious for 3 to four days.

During the fast patients are encouraged to move a lot in the open, like hiking, and every day there should be some guided exercise with a physiotherapist or a massage for people with back problems.

There are many more possibilities to help a body detoxify, for instance by dry brushing the whole skin except the face with a soft brush of organic material for 5 to ten minutes in the morning before taking a shower. This will take away the old cells of the outer layer and speed up the regeneration of new and healthy skin cells. Special bath therapies with herbal extracts can be applied regularly for people with metabolic problems or joint pain.

During siesta time a little bag filled with flowers and hay from the mountains can be placed on the digestive organs after the bag has been heated in hot steam for half an hour. This so-called hay sack can stay there for half an hour or longer, and it helps to soothe the liver and intestinal tract.

After the fasting procedures the cleansing process can be continued with herbal therapies for the main detoxifying organs liver and kidneys. We use Chinese herbal formulas or herbal teas, which can augment the liver metabolism and the gall flux. This regimen also helps the kidneys to eliminate substances from the blood and excrete them with the urine.

This is necessary for persons who tend to have oedema, and retain water in their body that has to be got rid of.

If there are real liver problems the long time consequences for this person should be considered. As the liver is not only the main detoxifying organ of the body but also some kind of chemical laboratory for the metabolism of proteins, fatty acids and carbohydrates, it should get all the help possible to enable a normal function.

We know what will be the consequences of impaired liver metabolism from people with liver cirrhosis whose brain functions in the end suffer greatly, as ammonia cannot be eliminated properly.

Liver cirrhosis can end up as liver cell carcinoma, or life-threatening bleeding can occur from varicose veins in the oesophagus or stomach. Therefore it is important to be aware of the possibilities we have for the prophylactic treatment of liver related problems with homeopathic remedies or Chinese medicine.

If we choose fasting as our initial cleansing regimen, we can begin with a fast of 10 to 14 days. Vegetable juices containing red beets, carrots, celery and a raw potato are recommended for that purpose.

The herbal tea during that time can contain liver related herbs like Carduus marianus, i.e. milk thistle, which helps with the liver cell metabolism, birch leaves, dandelion root and raspberry leaves. There are also Ayurvedic preparations such as Liv 52® that can help after breaking the fast.

Later the respective liver diet with food of high quality, preferably organically grown and plenty of antioxidants is essential to help that organ regain its function, which may have been impaired by environmental toxins or a specific virus such as one of the Hepatitis viruses or the Epstein Barr virus.

Treatment with homeopathy

In the field of homoeopathy there are even more possibilities to treat specific diseases, as the method of diluting and potentizing a substance by vigorous shaking can change the character of a remedy considerably. When this is done in steps of ten, that means one part of the substance is mixed with nine parts of water or a liquid containing alcohol, or do it with milk sugar, we get D-potencies as a result.

In steps of a hundred it will yields C-potencies. We used both possibilities and saw good results in either case, especially in the treatment of young children who were suffering from allergies or constant virus-induced catarrhs.

So why is this form of diluting and shaking necessary at all if you can use undiluted substances as well? The answer is very simple, because many substances, used in homeopathy, would be much too strong or poisonous if they were used in a concentrated form. Besides that homeopathic medications, which have been potentized, act differently from the same substance in a concentrated form.

If you need plenty of magnesium it is expedient to give both forms, for instance the concentrated magnesium orotate together with the homeopathic form of magnesium.

The homeopathic form is responsible for the dynamics and helps to absorb the concentrate for better usage in the organism. That can be helpful in case of muscle cramps.

But it becomes really interesting with substances, which are too poisonous to be used as a concentrate such as snake poisons. They have turned out to be very useful if applied in a homeopathic form. The Asian cobra for instance, called Naja tripudians, is a valuable remedy for people with heart problems, such as bad circulation because of coronary problems. It can even be helpful after a heart attack due to infarction. We used that in many cases in the diluted (potentized) form as D12 or higher, and had less ailments and relapses of the disease, while patients claimed to feel much better.

It is a similar story with the poison of the Brasilian snake Lachesis muta (bushmaster), the concentrated poison may easily kill a human being, but the diluted form can be used for numerous ailments. The feeling of constriction is a key symptom, which can appear as angina pectoris, angina tonsillaris or menopause symptoms and many others.
Constantin Hering gave a detailed description of the symptoms after he had been bitten by a bushmaster and barely survived. While he was in a delirium his wife had written down her observations, and later on they put together all the symptoms.

Many substance, which would be quite dangerous in the original form become valuable remedies with the homeopathic preparation. Even plants can be so poisonous as to kill people who try to make tea out of them. We had quite a few cases of teenagers who tried to become 'high' by drinking a concoction of the flowers of Angel's trumpet, belonging to the Datura species of the Solanacea family. Similarly used plants are Belladonna, which in a homeopathic form is a remedy for states of delirium or severe fever reaction with red and hot head, as can be seen in cases of infections with viruses or bacteria or because of other reasons.

Hyoscyamus is the third one in the family of Solanaceas, which can calm down people with severe unrest if given in a potentized form. They all contain alkaloids such as scopolamine, hyoscyamine and atropine.

In the undiluted native form they are anticholinergic substances, (that means antagonizing acetylcholine on nerve synapses), and thus weakening the parasympathetic nerve system. They produce symptoms of sympathetic preponderance such as photophobia, mydriasis (dilated pupils in the eye), hyperthermia and tachycardia, which can end up in delirium with possible consecutive death if the ingested dose was high enough.

We see here all the symptoms occurring also in connection with stress, where the sympathetic nerve excitation outweighs the parasympathetic.

But also these plants and similar ones can be used as a remedy in a diluted homeopathic form. By diluting and shaking them, (called potentizing), they become valuable calming and soothing remedies treating similar ailments as the concentrated drugs produce.

This is called the reverse action of homeopathy and constitutes an important principle that can be seen in all the substances used that way. It could be shown in rats that hazardous substances can be excreted faster with the help of such homeopathic preparations.

Another homeopathic specialty is the treatment with nosodes, such as the nosode hepatitis for liver problems.

As the term nosode may not be known to most people, we have to give a short explanation concerning the terminology.

Nosos in classical Greek means illness, and so nosodes are homoeopathic preparations manufactured from parts of diseased organs or microorganisms. They have been sterilised and diluted or rather brought into higher potency by diluting and vigorously shaking the substance. This creates something like a mini-vaccine in order to lead the organism on the way to healing.

The nosode is meant to activate the body for its self-restoration by leading the way and preventing an illness from becoming chronic. This is of great advantage, as every chronic process is much harder, sometimes impossible to cure.

Nosodes have been developed for many purposes, different organs and ailments. The author's experiences with nosodes during the past 30 years have been amazingly positive.

This applies especially to the treatment of little children, whose cures cannot be termed placebo effect, as critics of homoeopathy usually call every positive resonance of homoeopathic treatment.

Nosodes can even be used for diseases that actually had taken place quite some time ago, as the organism seems to have a keen memory for harmful events that leave toxins in the body. Sometimes the nosode triggers a crisis and replays the symptoms of the former disease in an amazing way.

This sounds frightening, but this happens only for a short time, and then after the targeted toxins have been eliminated the healing process can begin.

There are not only nosodes for the liver function, but also for the kidney and other organs that can be impaired by illness. It can also be necessary to apply nosodes of former diseases like scarlet fever or diphtheria, which can leave a heavy load of toxins in the system. Also the viruses mentioned in connection with the chronic fatigue syndrome such as EBV, Cytomegalo and all the others can be treated by applying the respective nosode.

The author had a very strong reaction herself when she applied the nosode of mumps for a disease that had taken place almost twenty years earlier. The name of that nosode is parotitis, which actually means inflammation of the salivary gland in front of the ear.

But the illness mumps (parotitis) can also go along with an inflammation of the pancreas as the respective virus also attacks that gland. This organ is important for the production of digestive enzymes and insulin and very vulnerable to toxins and stress.

In that case the nosode produced the same symptoms as the original illness, but they lasted only a few hours and never returned. Not even when a second dose of the same nosode parotitis was taken. The main detox-reaction seemed to have taken place after the first dose of that remedy. Many patients react in a similar way after nosodes are given.

As chronic diseases pose more and more problems, we tried a new approach of treatment by combining nosodes with Chinese medicine such as herbal formulas and got very rewarding results.

In order to understand how that works we have to make a short excursion into Chinese medicine in the next chapter.

The basics of Chinese medicine

The Chinese system tries to integrate body and mind, as every organ has a mental connection. The two forces of energy Yin and Yang are complementary and together they create life. Yin is the feminine principle and is passive, dark cold and moist. Yang is associated with the male principle and the hot, the light, the dry.

The five basic processes are the essence Jing, the spirit Shen, the Qi energy, the blood and the fluids. The Qi energy consists of several different parts with important functions:

Yuan Qi is the primordial Qi we received from our parents.

Gu Qi comes from our food, which the spleen uses to produce blood.

Kong Qi is received from the air we breathe, and it is associated with the lungs.

Zheng Qi is the energy that flows through the meridians and body organs.

Ying Qi helps to nourish our body with the food, air and water we ingest.

Wei Qi protects the surface of our body from the intrusion of exterior detrimental factors.

Qi can be deficient, sinking, stagnant or rebellious, thus creating different forms of ailments such as pain with stagnation, or vomiting with a rebellious Qi.

Blood can also be deficient or stagnant, heat in the blood can occur due to imbalances in the body or it can be a sign of deficient or inadequate Yin. This can frequently be seen in older people or individuals who burnt too much of their substance by overworking or stress.

The body has twelve major organs as storehouses of the body energies and fluids, they are equally divided into Yin and Yang organs.

The Yin organs are lungs, heart, liver, kidneys, spleen.

The pericardium is added, which is not an organ, but it enhances many of the heart functions; they all are called Zang organs.

The Yang organs are large intestine, small intestine, gallbladder, bladder and stomach, they receive and process the vital fluids. They are called Fu organs. The sixth one is the triple warmer or triple burner (San Jiao), and it is more an energy system, consisting of the upper, middle and lower burner.

The function of the yin organs

1. Lungs control vital Qi and respiration, are associated with skin and hair and house the physical part of the soul, Po. The complementary Yang organ is the large intestine.

2. Heart controls blood and blood vessels, is associated with face and tongue and houses the spirit, Shen. The complementary yang organ is small intestine.

3. Liver promotes flow of Qi, stores blood, is associated with the eyes and houses the ethereal soul, Hun. The complementary yang meridian is gallbladder.

4. Kidneys store the essence, Jing and rule growth, development and reproduction, control the brain,

marrow and bones and house the willpower, Zhi. The complementary yang meridian is bladder.

5. Spleen rules transformation and transportation of blood and vital fluids, moves Qi, holds the organs in place and houses the mind, Yi, it is associated with mouth, skin and limbs. The complementary yang organ is stomach.

6. Pericardium enhances several actions of the heart, the complementary yang organ is triple warmer.

The meridians

Meridians are non-physical energy channels that run along the surface of the body. They transport the energy through a network of pathways and connect the exterior with the interior.

Every meridian is in connection with a specific organ and there are certain invisible points, through which the energy can be accessed by acupuncture. This may become necessary if deficiency or stagnation of energy have become the cause of illness or pain.

The energy (Qi) circulates from one meridian to the next in a twenty-four hour cycle, so that every organ has a time of maximum energy.

This knowledge can be helpful in case some ailment becomes manifest at a certain time, such as awakening between 1 and 3 o'clock in the morning. As that is the time of maximum liver energy, the treatment should comprise liver remedies.

Meridians have a therapeutic relationship to Chinese herbs, as some herbs have a specific affinity for certain meridians and can be a powerful stimulant for the connected organ.

The causes of illness can be internal, that is emotional or psychological. They can also be external such as climatic in origin, as for instance caused by cold wind. External conditions may penetrate into the interior of the body and become more serious, that means they may have a complementary internal manifestation, as for instance exterior and interior wind. They can occur together, and so wind-cold as well as damp-heat can cause an illness by joint action. Wind is yang in nature and is characterized by its sudden onset and intensity of movement.

Cold is Yin in nature, and the symptoms can be those of a common cold beginning with chills, which later turn to fever. That is when the factor heat, which is yang in nature appears, which is accompanied by sweating or inflammation and swelling.

Dampness is Yin in nature, and is characterized by swelling and phlegm.

Dryness is Yang in nature and has loss of fluids, dry skin and hair or hacking cough.

Fire is yang in nature and shows extreme conditions of heat, often accompanied by emotional excesses, which are called inner fire and effect the stomach, lungs and liver.

The symptoms of illness have to be categorized in eight principle ways using Yin and Yang as starting points. They have to be identified according to the following qualities: internal-external, hot-cold and excess-deficiency. The therapy can comprise acupuncture and herbal therapy together with Qi gong (certain motions) or massage therapy.

Energy flow and psychosomatic illness

The main goal of Chinese medicine can be seen in the restoration of an unimpeded energy flow. Though the Chinese people thousands of years ago did not know what we know today, their point of view is quite close to the things we have learned as students when confronted with Einstein's formula $E = mc^2$.

It means that everything is energy, ruling our whole being, and there is plenty of emotional energy stored in our memory as pictures of our whole life, which can have a mighty influence on our behaviour. No matter if those pictures are consciously or subconsciously stored, they can change the whole function of our metabolism. Especially if traumatic incidents in connection with fear keep coming up with detrimental force, we get into a state of emergency.

There are so many people living in constant fear of failure in their jobs, of not being able to pay off the mortgage on their house, of becoming ill and dying or of authorities finding out that they did not pay their taxes, as they should have done. Some persons do not even know what they are afraid of, and still their anxiety is accompanying them for most of their lives. This can lead to a state of catatonic depression paralysing them and making them unable to lead a normal life.

Depression has been linked to the neurotransmitter serotonin, which in connection with dopamine seems to rule the state of our mind.

In this context we understand why antidepressants such as SSRIs (selective serotonin re-uptake inhibitors) have become such blockbusters, as for instance Prozac®. They prolong the time serotonin is effective, and thus artificially lighten up our mood.

For the treatment of psychosis the antagonistic action upon serotonin and dopamine receptors seems to play an important role, as for instance with the atypical antipsychotic drugs clozapine and olanzapine (Zyprexa®). But they cause serious side effects on metabolism, as patients gain weight, may become diabetics, and in elderly people stroke can be promoted.

As they are also effective for bipolar disease those drugs have also become blockbusters, and the sales of Zyprexa® alone in the United States were exceeding 2 billion dollars in 2010.

Anxiety and fear seem to be so common nowadays that no one seems to wonder how it can be that so many people need chemical help in order to keep their peace of mind.

Fear can influence us even on a sub-cellular level, that means the function of our cells including the mitochondria or even the DNA are impeded by our conscious and subconscious traumatic experiences.

Those events can have happened anytime in our life under different circumstances, though the most vulnerable time seems to be early childhood and the embryonic and foetal phase. At that point the child is forced to feel every emotion of his mother, and that may be fear, unhappiness or rejection of the pregnancy under unfortunate circumstances.

All the pictures and feelings of those events are stored lifelong and can be reactivated or triggered by a situation that has some resemblance to the former trauma, and thus brings up old painful memories.

In the process of reactivation the old trauma can totally determine our reaction, though the present situation may be in no way threatening. But the old negative memory can cause fear and determine our behaviour in a detrimental way, which causes us to react as if we were in an extremely stressful situation. From our feelings of fear we connect to the limbic system in our brain, a part of which is the hypothalamus. By activating our sympathetic nerve system it makes the adrenal medulla put out epinephrine (adrenalin).

The hypothalamus also sends out releasing factors, which cause the pituitary gland to put out ACTH (adrenocorticotropic hormone) and TSH (thyroid stimulating hormone) from the anterior part of the pituitary gland. This incites high levels of stress hormones in the adrenals, the thyroid and even the pancreas, where the hormone glucagon leads to a higher blood sugar level.

This cascade has high blood pressure, elevated heart rate and sweating as a consequence, because our stress hormones adrenaline (epinephrine) and cortisole have suddenly surged to high levels, whereas our digestive processes will be stopped. This vicious cycle can be endlessly perpetuated, and the body will not be allowed to come back to rest and normality. Under such unfortunate circumstances the whole metabolism will be altered, and recreational phases become virtually impossible. The consequence will be that the immune system suffers considerable damage, as cortisole interferes with B and T- lymphocytes and stops their forming and their function.

Thus all sorts of diseases can come up from allergies to autoimmune diseases or carcinomas, as the normal state of T-helper, T-suppressor and B- lymphocytes is out of balance, and the count of those cells can be greatly diminished. The consequences are dependant on the weak spot a certain individual may have or which organ is the weakest link in a chain and will suffer damage first.

In case of an autoimmune disease the thyroid gland is frequently the first organ to suffer, ending up in hypothyroidism due to Hashimoto's disease, which can be found out by searching for the specific TPO (thyroid peroxidase) antibodies. In some cases stress may lead to Grave's disease with hyperthyroidism and the specific TRAB (thyroid receptor antibodies). Many more illnesses can follow after the thyroid gets sick, as autoimmune processes rarely stop after affecting one organ.

Making the energy field visible

In energetic terms we can say in case of disease the energy field, which surrounds every living creature, suffers. Some people call that aura, which forms another invisible hull around the surface of our body on the outside. It can be made visible by placing a hand or a foot in an electromagnetic field and by taking a photo of that extremity. This is called Kirlian photography after The Russian engineer who established that method. This way of taking photos shows if a strong, normal energy field surrounds your hands and feet, or if there is deformation, weakening or a total absence of that field.

Now some people say those are all artefacts created by the external electro-magnetic field that is used for taking the photo. But how can it be that sometimes you see no aura around a hand or foot on one side, whereas the other side shows it under the same conditions of taking those photos. The former can be the case if a scar hinders the flow of energy, which seems to be led along the lines of the meridians found by the Chinese in ancient times.

What can be done in such a case to overcome the obstacle and make the energy flow again? The scar can be treated by an injection of a local anaesthetic, which alters the state of conductibility in tissues.

Thus the energy can overcome the obstacle and flow through the scar tissue. Then suddenly the energy field in the form of a corona comes up surrounding fingers and toes. The points emitting the radiation are the acupuncture points that are present on every extremity, they are especially numerous on fingers and toes. The localisation of the field showing deformation even gives hints as to which organ suffers and needs help.

We have seen the described phenomena many times by taking photos with the Kirlian method, and it can be considered as proven that bio currents and energy fields can be made visible that way. It can be shown that after an injection into and around scar tissue regularly a missing field comes up, and can be seen on the photo. This happens as the ion flow is changed by blocking Na-channels of cell membranes via injecting a local anaesthetic into scar tissue. This enables the bio current to flow more easily.

Without those bio-currents it would not be possible to write an electrocardiogram, an electroencephalogram or to see pictures created by MRI (magnetic resonance imaging), as all those techniques only make things visible that have always existed as an energetic field created by bio currents.

If we concede that traumatic energies can be stored in our memory like pictures on a film, the question is now how to blot out the detrimental influence that makes us behave as if being in a constant situation of emergency. That means stress hormones are activated every time a trigger situation arises, which reminds us of the former original incident, which really was causing fear. Some people live in a state of fear almost all their lives, as they always think of things that could go wrong, or they fear to be rejected, and that way tension and stress are perpetuated.

Another emotion that can severely harm the peace of mind is revengefulness and not being able to forgive, as this attitude leads to all kinds of detrimental consequences such as hatred and even actions of retaliation. These feelings even change the energy field and should also be taken care of in therapy.

Different forms of psychotherapy

Many different forms of psychotherapy have been tried to get people away from their harmful emotions starting from the early days of Freud till recently. Some therapists thought that bringing up events that had been partly buried, and talking about them in a therapeutic session would take the charge off the former traumatic situation. But in most cases that did not bring the desired relief. Whatever the method applied was called, we have seen people after all kinds of psychotherapies, but mostly they only learned to better cope with their situation. That means they learned to function in spite of the oppressive feelings, but in no way had the charge been taken off. It may even require more energy to apply the new technique of functioning in a way they had been taught in their therapeutic sessions, as the underlying cause remains.

We have seen some success by making people live through the feelings of the original trauma repeatedly. Sometimes this had to be done several times depending on the severity of the psycho trauma, which mostly had taken place in early childhood.
But it was painful to relive that situation, and it could take a long time to get rid of the charge. Therefore the therapy could go on for several years and the outcome was always uncertain.
Lately we came across a new approach called "The Healing Code", laid down in a book by Alexander Lloyd and Ben Johnson. It claims to help people become free of the influence

of old traumatic images, which can be triggered again and again by similar situations.

These old traumatic memories create a vicious cycle of stressful reactions making persons sick and desperate. According to the authors this can be changed by the method of the Healing Code, and even other ailments disappear by working according to that book. One of the authors is a former minister and now is a psychologist. He works by appealing to the faith of people handing over to God their hurt and bad memories, which create fear and tension, and by using healing energies.
They are directed to certain areas on the head where in Chinese medicine we find many important acupuncture points.

For Christians there exists another alternative as shown in the book "A More Excellent Way" by Henry Wright. It helps people to be restored to health by applying the principles of the Bible. Agnostic persons may not be able to go that way, as a person who does not believe in God can hardly accept His rules, otherwise they have to rethink their position. Nevertheless there have been amazing results, and that makes this book worth reading, thus everyone can select the way he wants to tackle his old traumatic memories.

Comparing the orthodox approach with Chinese therapies

Chinese medicine, as well as homeopathy, have always seen the energetic connections and considered life a phenomenon of flowing energy, which has to be restored in case of illness. The methods applied try to help the body without serious side effects.

In orthodox western medicine we seem to have accepted that almost all our so called remedies can also kill us, and nobody ever tells you there may be something wrong with your energy field. But when we look closer at orthodox medicine and consider the development of therapies during the past century, we see that a flood of chemical substances has come into use seemingly making all other natural or traditional therapies superfluous. But it has turned out in the meantime that life does not work that way. Often side effects made people sicker than they had been before or, as a result, the long time effects could not grant what had been promised. This has often been the case with chemotherapy for cancer, which prolongs people's lives for perhaps a few weeks for the price of heavy suffering.

Chinese medicine on the other hand works with energies flowing in the meridian system. They can be accessed at certain defined points with needles or with fingers, and thus stagnations or deficiencies be reverted back to normal.

Chinese herbs also seem to have an affinity to the energy system of the meridians, as certain herbs are mainly affecting special meridians where they influence the flowing energy.

Herbs can act warming in case of cold or Yin symptoms, and cooling for heat or Yang symptoms. False heat symptoms occur because of a Yin deficiency and therefore have to be treated differently, as the Yin deficiency has to be taken care of first. So if cold wind has invaded causing an illness, then warming the body and expelling the pathogen can help restore the body's balance back to health. If looking for a remedy that expels wind and is warm, as for the treatment of a common cold, you could use formulas, as given at the end of this book, containing some of the following herbs:

Cinnamon, Angelica dahurica, Ginger, Ledebouriella or Notopterygium.

Cooling heat in the blood or liver could be done with formulas containing Paeony root, Moutan bark root combined with liver remedies such as Bupleurum, Curcuma or Gentiana radix (root).

In cases of infectious diseases with heat (fever) remedies such as Fructus Forsythiae combined with folium(leaf) or radix (root) Isatidis can be of great help. This boosts the immune system and expels the pathogen, which means it gets rid of the symptoms and the virus.

It has turned out that many diseases that are due to imbalances in the body can be treated by Chinese medicine where the orthodox western approach is not very successful or the side effects of treatment make the patient sick in another way.

We will also give a list of Chinese herbs, which are contained in the formulas later in this book. But as they are potent remedies, they should only be applied under the supervision of a practitioner who knows how to handle those herbs.

In our experience it turned out to be quite a good combination to give nosodes to cleanse and Chinese herbs to build up new energies and substance.

This turned out especially advantageous in older patients, as we tend to lose more and more of our substance (yin) during the aging process. Although the aging process can vary in a broad range, according to the life someone has led, he or she can slow the process down considerably by omitting the worst mistakes that can be made when people are still young and presumably healthy.

Mistakes we will have to pay for

We will try to present a list of mistakes people make while they think they can afford to do so, because they feel strong and invincible.

The worst thing you can do for your body is smoking, with hundreds of toxic components in the tobacco smoke. Women especially pay a high price for this, as their aging process is much faster than it would be without that vice. Their skin becomes thin and vulnerable and full of wrinkles, but that is only the outside.

The inner surfaces like cell membranes and the inner layer of blood vessels degenerate and become rugged with plaques for both genders, and the consequences are thromboses, strokes, heart infarctions and other circulation problems.

If the second grave mistake is combined with smoking we get even worse results. The second fault is overeating, which due to lack of sufficient exercise leads to obesity, metabolic problems such as diabetes, sluggish digestion and problems with cholesterol, uric acid and the like.

Choosing the wrong food products such as an overload of sugar leads to deficiencies of necessary nutrients, so that the body never feels satisfied, and the craving for sugar increases. If the quality of nutrition is low, mostly the quantity becomes higher. In the course of time it can create a state where people permanently think they are hungry and eat more and more junk food because of that feeling.

Needless to say that obesity and metabolic problems will be the consequence.

The third grave mistake is drinking alcohol, and that not only damages the liver, but leads to a vicious cycle of malnutrition and vitamin deficits, especially of the B-group such as Pyridoxine (Vit.B6) or thiamine, which is Vitamin B1, both vitamins are necessary for the metabolism of the liver and the nerves.

We have to emphasize at this point that sugar and refined carbohydrates have no place in a healthy nutrition, as well as soft drinks, lots of coffee and strong black tea. All processed food like ready made meals or dressings, and all sorts of canned food should be omitted. Toxic chemicals for the household are to a large portion superfluous, as much as possible should be cleaned with neutral soap. Chemically cleaned clothes are a constant source of toxic components and should not be worn for some time after the cleaning process.

Food should be cooked fresh and not for several days in advance and then kept in the fridge or freezer, because the quality is inferior and gets less with warming.

Fresh raw food should also be present in our nutrition.

How nutrition can be improved

How then should proper nutrition be in order to contribute to our health?

For that purpose let us compare the normal western diet with the kind of nutrition that would be desirable. In the western diet, many people eat, more than 40% of their calorie intake is due to fats, mostly of the saturated type.

This is dangerous, because 1 gram of fat delivers 9 calories, which can lead to obesity and elevated LDL cholesterol. It would be more advisable to limit the fat intake to 15 to 20 percent of their calorie intake with a higher amount of vegetable oil.

Carbohydrates on the other hand deliver just 4 calories per gram, but they can cause diabetes, if a considerable part consist of sugar and white meal products. We should rather have more complex carbohydrates in our nutrition, which could be up to seventy percent.

Proteins yield the same number of calories as carbohydrates per gram, and they should not be predominantly of animal sources. On the whole it can be said that the LDL Cholesterol in relation to the HDL is raised with higher intake of saturated fats or trans fats.

The amount of fibres comes to about 10 to 15 grams, but should be three times that much, which would slow down the absorption of carbohydrates, and thus lead to lower blood sugar levels.

There are soluble and insoluble fibres, mostly of vegetable source. Both are necessary for our wellbeing, the soluble sort can be digested, the insoluble sort adds bulk to our bowel contents and enhances bowel movement.

The western diet leads to sluggish metabolism with problems for liver and bowels, because the amount of fibre is too low, and the amount of saturated fat is too high.

Apart from that a high portion of animal protein leads to a high probability of deposition of clogging material in blood vessels. It also causes putrid decomposition of protein in the large bowel, and thus an elevated rate of colonic cancer.

It has been proven on the other hand that proteins of vegetable source, as contained in nuts and seeds or green vegetables, are readily available and do not lead to such hazardous consequences. Besides that meat contains lots of phosphorus, and thus in the long run depletes the body of calcium, as the two elements have to be balanced.

This can lead to detrimental diseases like osteoporosis or osteomalacia as a consequence. In case of osteomalacia the soft structures of the bone cannot incorporate enough minerals and start to deform.

Though we often heard from our parents that meat is necessary to build up proteins in our body, it can be shown that vegetable protein is in no way inferior to animal protein. Soybeans, for instance, contain about the same composition of amino acids as beef.

From all this we can see that it is not necessary to eat meat, on the contrary, it is advantageous for people's health to eat vegetarian meals. But if someone does not want to renounce completely, he should at least limit the meat intake to twice a week and seek to buy good quality.

Under health aspects vegetarian nutrition has the advantage that people do not tend to overeat, and that the consumption of raw fresh food has shown the best results in respect to longevity.

With lots of fresh salads and fruit in combination with wholemeal products all the necessary nutrients such as minerals, enzymes and vitamins, as well as flavonoids and other plant products, which act as antioxidants are amply available.

That way we have less clogging up of our system and better oxygenation of the tissues, which leads to better health, whereas degenerative processes can be kept at bay.

If we want to express that in numbers, it would mean that the amount of fat in a healthy nutrition should not be more that 20% of the overall calories, but the intake of complex carbohydrates should be much higher, namely 60 to 70 percent. Protein comprising about 15% should be mostly of vegetable origin, because it is more readily available and does not lead to the production of noxious substances like scatole, indol, putrescine or cadaverine in the bowel. Exactly this is what happens with an overload of animal proteins, especially red meat, which can promote atherosclerosis, as we already discussed in connection with carnitine.

Fibres are very important for our bowel system, and our nutrition should contain about 50 grams of those substances, which are present in most vegetables and grains. Soybeans and other legumes such as peas and lentils are very recommendable as they contain valuable proteins and fibres.

This would be a diet leading to an increased flexibility and permeability of the membranes of our cells, thus creating an augmented energy flow adding to wellbeing and longevity.

As it should be the goal to get older without suffering from the ailments of aging, unimpeded energy flow through those membranes is essential.

Allergies, incompatibilities and homoeopathy

But what can be done if you are sick, even as a young individual, because you have been allergic from childhood on, suffering from eczema, asthma or even an auto-immune disease? In that case we will really have to take a close look at all the circumstances, because the reasons can differ on a large scale from one individual to the other.

Often inherent genetic traits predispose an individual to be highly allergic to all kinds of pollen, cat's hair or even certain foods. First thing with food allergies should be to find out, if the allergies against certain vegetables still persist, when only organically grown vegetables are consumed. Frequently that will not be the case, and despite incompatibility for cows' milk it will often be possible to consume goat milk products.

Sometimes allergies appear at an age when no one has thought of it any more. The author had a patient well in her forties who had developed food incompatibilities to such an extent that she often did not know what she could eat at all. Close questioning of the patient brought forth the following: The German women had spent several years in South America, and had in the course of time suffered from tropical diseases such as malaria. The diseases had been treated with synthetic medication and on the surface she had been cured. But after that the allergies started and got worse after her return to Germany.

When this woman came to our private clinic as a patient for several weeks, we began with a cleansing program for liver and kidneys starting with a two weeks' fast. Then herbal remedies for her liver were the next step of our therapy, but no progress with the food allergies was to be seen.

Now the nosodes for the tropical diseases were chosen as therapy, and after 6 weeks' therapy with nosodes and further cleansing, she for the first time ate some of her former allergens, but in the organically grown version.

This time nothing happened, she was not reacting to these vegetables that a few weeks before had caused so many problems. This seemed almost miraculous, especially as the allergies did not come back later. But she had changed her nutrition in the sense that she only consumed organically grown vegetables and regularly went on a cleansing fast.

Allergies in children often pose problems because they can appear very early in life, as genetic reasons seem to play a major role.

But it must never be forgotten that environmental toxins can pass through the placenta and are handed from mother to child during pregnancy, and even stress during pregnancy can influence the child's allergic disposition.

In cases of health problems during early childhood it always pays to scrutinise the mother and find out what kind of toxins she may have passed on. It is also important what conditions the mother was living in during the time of pregnancy.

The author once had a patient with mercury intoxication from her numerous amalgam fillings, from which she had plenty of health problems. Her small boy of 11 months was also sick most of the time either with virus infections or skin allergies or both at the same time.

Therefore we decided to begin a therapy for the excretion of heavy metals with a chelating agent, in this case DMSA in the form of capsules.

After the mother responded well to the therapy, we tried a mild therapy with the same substance, but in lower dosage for the child.

The boy got the lowest dose available, and within 4 weeks we could see a turn for the better as his skin notably improved, and the virus infections cased. Both patients got mineral supplements with the therapy and herbal support, the mother even went on a short fast to stabilise her condition.

Miasma and homeopathic therapy

That leads us to another aspect of inherited diseases, the so-called miasma. The term miasma is classical Greek and means pollution. The German Physician Samuel Hahnemann who created the system of homeopathy, used this term back in the 18th century, not meaning pollution of the environment, but of the inner parts of our body.

He found out that people in whose family there had been severe illnesses like Syphilis, Gonorrhoea or Psora,(that means skin problems), there could be consequences from residues of those diseases in later generations.

Therefore inherited weaknesses of certain kinds such as the nervous system, bones, skin and so on could have their origin therein. He called these miasmata (plural of miasma), and created the nosodes Luesinum, Medorrhinum and Psorinum as remedies against these inherited weaknesses.

Everyone of these nosodes has specific features according to the miasma.

Luesinum is the remedy against destructive features, which affect nerves and bones, with the worst symptoms at night. Those persons generally feel worse near the sea and suffer from a weak nerve system, which is called neurasthenic constitution.

Whereas Medorrhinum is characterised by symptoms of unrest and inflammation with the worst time during the day, while they feel better near the sea.

Psora is sluggish in character, it is mostly needed in connection with skin symptoms, such as eczema of an inherited nature. Those three classic nosodes have turned out to be very important in cases with a hereditary component.

Another nosode, which was introduced later by one of Hahnemann's disciples, is Tuberculinum. This became one of the most important homoeopathic remedies for children with allergies or suffering from frequent virus infections. The nosode Tuberculinum is indicated for people with tendencies to fever and a rash and timid temperament.

The susceptibility for infections is frequent in families with a history of tuberculosis in one of the former generations.

Many children and adults in Europe after World War1 and World War2, were suffering from malnutrition, therefore tuberculosis was very frequent. The closer in time the illness has occurred in the family, the more intense the disposition for the respective child, that means the mother's disease counts more than the grandmother's.

So it makes sense to try the nosode Tuberculinum for the mentioned inherited dispositions as therapy. Children with allergies or persons with severe rheumatic diseases, which frequently have genetic reasons as well, could profit from the application of all the miasmatic remedies.

Our treatment with those nosodes was often successful when applied to children with asthma. They should be given together with homoepathic remedies such as Cuprum aceticum, Spongia, Pulmonaria or Chinese herbal formulas. We had quite a few cases where the therapy of asthma with beta-mimetic drugs or cortison could be ended that way. We often used the aforementioned nosode Tuberculinum for children, even if an individual turned out to be tuberculin-negative. That means the person has never had contact with the actual bacillus, as shown in the skin testing.

But it could well be a reason for illness because of an inherent genetic trait in the family. One parent or grandparent may have suffered from that disease, and in one of the following generations this would be manifested as nervous instability or susceptibility for infections.

Mostly the homeopathic therapy of children showed good results, often in combination with nosodes.

Also paediatric diseases such as scarlet fever, measles or mumps can lead to toxic residues in the body, which can successfully be taken care of with nosodes and other homoeopathic remedies or in combination with Chinese herbs.

Nowadays many children never get those classic diseases any more, because they are vaccinated at an early age against all those illnesses. Now the question arises, if vaccination can also lead to toxic residues.

There have been controversies about the proper use of vaccination for quite a while. Most vaccines containing six or seven components are given to children at an early age, and that can easily be a stress factor for the immune system of young children. In our experience the treatment with the respective nosodes after vaccination rendered very positive results, whereas the protection created by the vaccine was in no way diminished. By applying nosodes to children who had reacted in an unfavourable way to vaccination with six or more ingredients we often saw a great deal of improvement, especially for skin problems. It could also result in more stability for the immune system, so we can say that less infect susceptibility and decreasing allergic manifestations could be seen after using nosodes of vaccination as treatment.

Attention Deficit Hyperactivity syndrome

Children with Attention Deficit Hyperactivity Syndrome could also profit from this therapy, as they become more stable in their reactions. We have found that this disease mostly arises from a combination of several factors from within and from outer sources.

Those sources could be extensive vaccination at an early age together with a flood of stimulants. These could be, television, computer games or internet activities. Other factors could be faulty nutrition with lack of minerals and trace elements together with residues of toxic substances, and often some conflict in the family is present as well.
In all these cases a miasma as a hereditary factor could be in the background making treatment with Medorrhinum, Luesinum or Tuberculinum necessary.

The orthodox treatment is with Methylphenidate (Ritalin®), a substance, which is related to amphetamines.
It is a so-called re-uptake inhibitor for nor-epinephrine and dopamine, which act as neuro-transmitters in our brain, and it prolongs the action of adrenergic substances.

That way it acts as a psycho-stimulant and increases the activity of the central nervous system, which can become hazardous. It is not amazing in that context that statistics show a higher rate of delinquency in individuals who had been treated with Methylphenidate (Ritalin®).

When parents are not willing to have their child treated with this substance, we try to offer alternatives. These could be nosodes and other homeopathic remedies, often in combination with Chinese herbal formulas, as well as trace elements, minerals and a different form of nutrition.

In most cases the whole family has to be treated, as often the reasons for that syndrome have their roots not in the child alone, but the entire family shows hidden problems.

Autoimmune diseases with possible ways of treatment

A special problem of our time arises with the increase of autoimmune diseases. As they can cover a broad field, it is not easy to find a common denominator for this kind of illness. It seems to be a long way from the autoimmune inflammation of the thyroid gland to an illness like multiple sclerosis. But they all have one common trait by building up antibodies against the body's own tissues.

Those antibodies can be thyroid receptor antibodies (TRAB) resulting in Grave's disease with hyperthyroidism, TPO (thyroid-peroxidase) antibodies in Hashimoto's disease with hypothyroidism with consecutive slowing down of the metabolism as visible in weight gain. Antibodies against nerve sheaths can also be found, resulting in multiple sclerosis. The body's own regulation seems to be completely out of balance to be in a position of attacking its own structures.

If it takes place in the kidneys the autoimmune process gradually destroys the functional parts of that filtering organ, the so-called glomeruli. They are little capillary coils, which produce the primary urine. If those capillary loops degenerate, as can happen through an autoimmune nephritis, the patient in the end has to be treated by dialysis.
These autoimmune processes can take place in almost every organ from kidney and liver to joints, connective tissue or the nervous system.

Autoimmune diseases all have in common that the immune system destroys the body's own organs through a specific form of inflammation. This can happen through the action of T-lymphocytes or by producing antibodies.

Probably our unhealthy lifestyle has a great part in the development of this kind of disease, bcause the toxins in our environment play an important role.

Apart from that autoimmune phenomena mostly have a strong psychological component, going back to former traumata and problems that could not be solved. Many people are not aware of those phenomena, because they emerge from the subconscious, but they still can evoke strong reactions such as autoimmune diseases.

Another aspect seems to be important, especially in connection with nerve related phenomena and processes that take place in joints and connective tissue.

Patients with those ailments often have a history of suppressing fever reactions during virus infections. Instead of staying at home with an infectious disease caused by a virus, they rather take tablets like Aspirin or antibiotics and go to work. Thus their body cannot deal with the infection but will keep it for a while in a suppressed state leaving a lot of toxins in the system.

In the end that can culminate in misled immune reactions such as autoimmune diseases, if this behaviour is the usual way of handling febrile infections. People who think they are indispensible tend to act that way, and therefore they have to go to work in order to keep the business from collapsing. This behaviour shows compulsive traits, and is mostly far from reality.

Orthodox medicine acknowledges that virus infections are a probable cause for diseases like multiple sclerosis, as viruses can stay in the body for a long time or even lifelong and change the balance of the immune system.

This is known of the hepatitis C virus and many others. In such cases we try an intense regimen with fasting, new dietary schedules and therapies with virus nosodes and corresponding herbs, Chinese formulas and homoeopathic support. But it should never be forgotten to take care of the psychological component as well.

That way we have seen a number of cases that had quite a favourable outcome. Sometimes it takes a long time to see results, but mostly it pays off to stick to the therapies for several months.

As we could see autoimmune diseases have their roots in toxins we had not got rid of, because we did not realise how detrimental our behaviour has been. This can act together with a hereditary trait and traumatic experiences with unresolved problems.

Comparison between homeopathy and Chinese medicine

These examples have basically shown that the homeopathic approach is a very individual one. It has to rely on intense questioning of the patient in order to find out the symptoms of his ailments, and to determine his constitution and get a family history. All this plays an important role in order to find out, which factors may be causative for the present disease.

On the other hand the approach in Chinese medicine has also clear regulations as how to diagnose and treat a patient. Besides the anamnesis, that is the intense questioning of the patient, a close inspection and palpation of the body with an emphasis on the tongue and pulse diagnosis will follow.

Then everything is brought into the order of eight principle ways, (Ba Gang), according to Yin-Yang, internal-external, excessive-deficient and hot-cold discernment.

Those symptoms determine the treatment with acupuncture, Chinese herbal formulas, massages or Chi Gong and Tai Chi (motion therapy).

The blood and energy-flow should be unimpeded, because stagnation leads to pathological symptoms like pain.

All major organs are in connection with certain energies that have to be restored if they are deficient. Those energies rule perceptions like hearing (kidney) or seeing (liver).

The Chinese approach is consistent in itself, though quite different from the western system of orthodox medicine, and it can be integrated into a holistic approach and combined with other therapies like homeopathy. You could even say that the two methods are complementary. Building up energies works best with Chinese formulas after the cleansing of inherent organ deficiencies has been brought about with nosodes and constitutional remedies, as done in homoeopathy.

Different diseases and comparison of treatment

In the next section we will deal with special conditions, for which we will give advice in alphabetical order according to the methods and regimens previously mentioned.

Acne and other skin problems

Acne and other skin related diseases under a holistic approach are not considered to be local problems. Therefore they cannot be cured by a local treatment with ointments alone.

The skin is a complicated structure with several layers and interspersed glands for sweat and lubrication with fatty substances, and we have to acknowledge that it also is an organ of excretion.

Sometimes it is called the third kidney, because in cases of kidney damage substances like uric acid are excreted through the skin and can be seen there as shimmering crystals on the surface; that happened quite often in times when dialysis was not available everywhere. So the skin transports toxic substances to the surface, when there is a lot of waste that has to be removed. This can happen with kidney malfunction or when the liver detoxifying capacity is impaired.

This can be due to illness or a simple overload with toxins through bad conditions in the environment or bad eating habits that have lasted for some time.

The skin can show all kinds of alterations from acne to derangement of pigmentation or allergic manifestations. In those cases it would not make sense to only treat the skin. The underlying problems, like clogged up metabolism with an overload of toxins the liver could not cope with, should be tackled instead. Chances are that the skin then will clean up as a consequence.

Mostly that happens without any external application of disinfectant therapy in the case of acne, or cortisone ointments in cases of allergies.

In order to help these organs with the excretion of waste products we can begin with a cleansing fast for 10 to 14 days and proceed with support for the liver. There are liver supporting herbs in Chinese medicine as well as classic European plants that can be used for that purpose. We will give a survey of herbs later.

In most cases the nutrition has to be changed, and all the fatty and sweet things that today are in broad use have to be given up. Instead the food has to consist of lots of fresh fruit and vegetables, cleansing herbal tea for the liver and a sufficient amount of free liquid. But the liquid should not consist of coffee or black tea.

Useful supplements of vitamins like Niacin and vitamin A can be tried, and external cleansing masks with fresh cucumbers or oat bran cooked for a short time in water will be helpful.

Carbuncles with pus can be treated with little bags containing cooked linseed or a paste made of goldenseal powder. Trace elements for the immune system such as Zinc and Manganese should not be forgotten.

Allergies

As we continue with the letter A, we come to allergies, which have increased on a large scale during the past decades. With very small children we see lots of allergies in connection with their skin so that often cows' milk will not be tolerated without risking serious conditions of the skin or allergies of the respiratory tract.

First thing to do should be to substitute goats' milk for cows' milk, and in most cases it will be tolerated. Breastfeeding seems to be superior to formula feeding and with allergic children vaccination should be undertaken carefully, not to give too many components at the same time.

In quite a number of cases the nosode Tuberculinum in a high potency can help to stabilize the immune system. If a child persists to have allergic symptoms like asthma or eczema homeopathic remedies like Cuprum aceticum for asthma or Calcium carbonicum for the skin can be tried, in order to avoid potentially harmful remedies like cortisone or beta mimetic drugs that weaken the immune system. The latter can lead to irritating states of tachycardia.

Allergies may develop at any age, and it is not only sensitisation to food, dust mites, pollen and animals' hair that cause the most problems, but the thousands of newly created chemical components that are present almost everywhere in the environment.

The most important advice for allergic people would be to make everything fresh and not to buy any processed or preserved food, as it usually contains preservatives and the like. It is important to prevent being confronted with potentially harmful preservatives, colourings or other chemical components that may act as allergens.

Living in a city with a lot of traffic constitutes the risk of having contact with all the toxic ingredients of automobile fumes and micro dust as of Diesel engines that in it self is a risk of sensitisation. It could be shown that children living on streets with heavy traffic had a higher rate of sensitisation to pollen than children living in streets with little traffic. The micro particles from automobiles, especially Diesel engine exhaust seem to beset pollen and make them more aggressive causing greater sensitisation.

The so-called food allergies in many cases are not real allergies, but incompatibilities, which do not show the classical pattern of antibodies that will react with antigens. In most cases we will not find antibodies, even by taking blood samples for tests like RAST, (radio-allergo-sorbent test).

This is a search for specific IG_E antibodies in order to determine to what substance a person is allergic.

As for incompatibilities it can be quite challenging to find out which food a certain person is intolerant to. This can be done with a very simple diet of rice and a few vegetables. Then things are gradually added one by one every third day.

That is necessary because it mostly takes longer than 24 hours for a reaction to come up when something incompatible has been eaten. Thus the food component that does not agree can be found out in the course of time. Nevertheless many food intolerances seem to be not a primary thing, but the consequence of other disturbances that happened through toxins, as the case of the woman and the tropical diseases on page 116 clearly demonstrates.

Therefore an environment with clean air and organically grown food is highly recommended to keep allergies at bay, even if there is a genetic disposition. The most common foods, which can cause incompatibilities are shown in the following list.

Eggs, milk, nuts and peanuts, fish, shrimps, lobster, gluten, which will be found in many grain products, especially when made of wheat flour, frequently cause problems. But also citrus fruits and many other fruits can be a source of incompatibility.

In case of a gluten problem rice, corn, buckwheat and millet should be used instead of wheat, gluten free bread is now available almost everywhere.

Sometimes it takes a long time to find out, which food components are the ones that cause an allergy. In lucky cases it can happen that through cleansing and changing the eating habits those food incompatibilities disappear.

Allergy testing for substances such as pollen or animals' hair is normally done with the prick test on the inside of patients' arms. It yields reliable results as to which agent is responsible for the stuffed nose or watering eyes.

But when it comes to therapy things are not so easy, as the desensitising therapy with injections in increasing doses for a long time does not always lead to a fortunate outcome. We have seen cases where an allergy against grass pollen might have gone, but other allergies have come up instead, or the patient develops food intolerances that have not been there before the injection therapy.

So in cases of children with allergies we mostly try the homoeopathic approach, before anything like injections are started. In most cases the response to those remedies is fairly good.

A list of homeopathic remedies will be given at the end of the book.

Fasting can also be a regimen to for people with allergies. Besides that calcium, magnesium and trace elements seem to have a stabilising effect on allergic patients.

Atherosclerosis

The next important question is what can be done to prevent atherosclerosis, because that leads to many consecutive diseases such as strokes, heart infarction or losing a leg.

This is not uncommon in smokers who ruined the walls of their arteries by confronting them with all the toxic substances that are contained in tobacco smoke, which can also have lung cancer as a consequence. So we have good reasons not to smoke, but that alone may not be enough, though it is a prerequisite of preventing atherosclerosis and all the following illnesses.

But there is much more that can and should be done not to fall prey to the aforementioned diseases.

It is well established that the beginnings of atherosclerosis go way back into early youth, so it would be of great advantage if children could get some healthy meals at school and learned how to prepare them. Then they could find out that they really taste good. It is essential to show children that there are alternatives to the kind of junk food that is so high in their favour.

Wholemeal products are as important as are fresh salads and vegetable dishes, so that meat will not be considered indispensible for every day meals. Fresh fruit should be eaten regularly, and soft drinks like cola or lemonades should not be the normal beverage.

Fish with the omega-3 fatty acids is more recommendable than meat, and many vegetables such as soybeans contain valuable protein.

As the common western diet also contains too much fat chemically called triglycerides, which means, every molecule of glycerine has three fatty acids bound to it. There are long chain fatty acids and short chain ones, they can be of a saturated type or unsaturated, which means having at least one double bond between the carbon atoms. They turn into saturated ones by taking up a hydrogen atom.

Essential fatty acids cannot be built up in our metabolism, they are of an unsaturated type, and can be taken up out of vegetable oil or fish oil.

They act in a protective way on the internal walls of blood vessels, and they can counteract all kinds of inflammations.

Essential fatty acids are necessary for our wellbeing, basically they consist of linolenic (an omega-3) and linoleic (an omega-6) fatty acid, leading to whole cascades of metabolic products in both lines, which are acting in an antagonistic way to each other.

As we already discussed earlier the saturated variety of fatty acids is the dangerous type, because it poses many problems to our metabolism, as it increases the LDL cholesterol.

From the uptake of fats with our food it is quite a long way through our digestive tract. Bile acids help in the processing of dietary fats by forming micelles, (that means smaller droplets that can be more easily digested.) After that the lipase of the pancreas separates the fatty acids from the glycerine. Then the fatty acids have to be digested into smaller molecules, called acetyl groups. In that process we get lots of sour products that can further condense to longer toxic products such as acetone.

This happens frequently in the diabetic patient whose metabolism is out of balance. But normally the acetyl groups are processed in the citric acid cycle where they are used to create energy.

It takes a lot more oxygen to process fat molecules in the metabolism than it would take to digest carbohydrates. That means the so-called respiratory quotient (RQ) is not good for fats. The respiratory quotient is defined as the ratio of carbon dioxide produced, to the volume of oxygen that is needed to oxidise a substance. The oxidation of carbohydrates results in a RQ of 1, whereas fat has a RQ of 0.7 and protein of 0.9. That means more oxygen is necessary to metabolize fats than proteins or carbohydrates. This may become important under fasting conditions when after a few days the carbohydrate reserve, which is stored in the liver in the form of glycogen, has been used up, and the body starts burning its fat reserves. Another fact is that fats contain more calories per gram than carbohydrates or proteins do.

1 gram of fat contains 9 K calories, whereas carbohydrates or proteins contain only 4. So the intake of triglycerides should be limited in order not to use up more oxygen than is absolutely necessary, and to prevent acid-forming processes in the course of burning fats.

Apart from that fat is a heavy carrier of calories. People who are overweight and have a breathing problem like COPD (chronic obstructive pulmonary disease) can run into serious trouble when living on a diet high in fat calories.

When it comes to preventing atherosclerosis, nutrition and exercise are the two dominant factors. Not smoking is surely as important because of the numerous toxic substances in tobacco smoke.

High cholesterol is also a risk factor that should be kept well under control. Eating plenty of fresh fruit and vegetables has turned out to be helpful for that task. But it should never be forgotten that the cholesterol levels are mostly genetically determined. It may be possible that one person can eat eggs every day, and the other cannot do so without having his cholesterol in a high range.

But nevertheless it pays to keep cholesterol, especially the LDL, and triglycerides at a low level, as well as homocystein, lipoprotein a, c-reactive protein and ADMA, which are also risk factors for atherosclerosis, as we have already discussed in the respective chapter.

There are more predisposing factors that have to be considered in the prevention of atherosclerosis. One of them is high blood pressure, which plays an equally important role in that respect. High blood pressure not only damages the heart but also the inner layers of the arteries by creating minor lesions on which the deposition of fatty material can begin. This is mostly accompanied by inflammation of the inner walls.

In the end this can lead to a state where the lumen of that artery is narrowed considerably. In the coronary arteries this may lead to the consequence of heart infarction.

Inflammatory processes of blood vessels seem to play a certain role in the obliteration of arteries, for instance in vasculitis, which is an inflammation of the inner layers of an artery, pertaining to an autoimmune process.

As already mentioned autoimmune processes have increased during the past few decades. This can take place in almost every organ and part of the body.

Though the renal arteries may be concerned by this inflammation, impairment of renal function can go unnoticed for quite a number of years. Sometimes it is manifested during pregnancy, as so many factors change in body function under the influence of a different hormonal balance. We will discuss this further in the chapter on high blood pressure.

Arthritis

We come to the next challenging subject, and that is arthritis. There are different types such as osteoarthritis meaning a process of degenerative changes in joints due to wearing off of joint cartilage. The surface of all joints is covered by cartilage composed of a hyaline structure, which is interspersed with cells called chondrocytes.

The regenerative capacity of cartilage is poor, because it contains no blood vessels. In the course of time and with sports or accidents that damage the joints the cartilage deteriorates, and motion will become more and more painful. At the age of 50 about 10% of the population suffer from osteoarthritis and every decade this number becomes greater, so by the age of 80 it is almost 100%.

Lots of disabilities are due to osteoarthritis, and the only question is, what to do not to be struck by that disease unseemly early. There are preparations of chondroitin and hyaluronic acid available that can be taken orally or as an injection in the case of hyaluronic acid. Another substance that has a favourable effect on joint metabolism is green lip muscle from New Zealand.

The problems that arise from the inflammatory form of arthritis (rheumatoid arthritis) are even worse and can happen at an early age, because it is not a degenerative process that takes place. The inflammatory form is a destructive autoimmune disease that has a genetic base.

It can be made worse by other forms of inflammation in the body, such as infected teeth or chronic tonsillitis. Virus infections can also be a promoting agent for inflammations.

In orthodox medicine the therapy of autoimmune diseases consists mostly of suppressing the inflammation by methotrexate or other drugs such as cortisone designed to modify the immune response.

It has been found in recent years that the cytokine Tumour Necrosis Factor plays a key role in the development of many chronic inflammatory diseases. Cytokines are small proteins molecules for signalling in intermolecular communication, and they have an immune-modulating role.

Tumor Necrosis Factor is an important component in chronic inflammatory processes with autoimmune character such as psoriatic arthritis, ankylosing spondylitis, rheumatoid arthritis, and also Crohn's disease.

Antagonists against the Tumour Necrosis Factor have been developed, such as the T N F inhibitors Adalimumab, Etanercept and Infliximab (Remicade®).

These substances significantly reduce inflammatory symptoms, improve function, reduce damage done to afflicted joints, and give patients a better quality of life.

On the other hand those therapies bring about the risk of reactivating tuberculosis or they may be leading to the development of lympho-proliferative diseases, lupus like skin symptoms, demyelination or reactivation of multiple sclerosis. Therapies should not be applied within 10 years after cancer treatment or during pregnancy.

These substances are all monoclonal antibodies that have been artificially created. Infliximab is not purely human, but it is a chimera, being partly of murine (mouse) origin. Because of that, in a small percentage there may be a reaction to the foreign component, either on the skin or more generalized.

But nevertheless we have seen cases of severe ankylosing spondylitis (Bechterev's disease) with excruciating pain in the spine, which had become almost rigid at that time, where Infliximab (Remicade®) was the only remedy that brought some relief.

If the ileo-sacral joint is inflamed in the course of that disease, other joints will mostly follow. There is no real cure for that illness, which is genetically determined, so help means only to alleviate symptoms.

There exists a certain antigen, which is seen in connection with ankylosing spondylitis, and that is the HLA B27. It is present in every cell, its genetic information is located on chromosome 6, and it ist is present in 97% of patients with ankylosing spondylitis. But only a small portion of people who carry that gene will develop that crippeling form of spondylitis.

With biological treatment of arthritis we had favourable results with juice fasting and treatment with natural vitamin E, Calcium, trace elements and herbal or homoeopathic medication with nosodes. Also the Chinese form of treatment with formulas such as Clematis and Stephania showed good results. But all those therapies have to be selected individually in order to be able to meet the exact requirements of the patient.

The administration of the enzyme bromelain, out of pineapples can also help to reduce the swelling and the pain in rheumatoid arthritis. As the enzyme is destroyed by cooking it will be of advantage to eat plenty of raw pineapple. Certain sprouts such as lucerne (alfalfa), and cleansing herbs like chaparral or cats' claws will also act favourably on arthritis.

In severe cases a diet rich in alkaline foods like fruits and vegetables, nuts and seeds instead of meat, as well as omitting large quantities of coffee and strong black tea is advisable. Citrus fruits, except grapefruit are not recommended, they do not seem to act favourably in most cases of arthritis.

Mustard plasters can be applied in case of osteoarthritis and poultices with herbs such as Slippery Elm bark, Cayenne, or Goldenseal can be used in rheumatoid arthritis, as they will alleviate inflammation and pain.

Deficiency of trace elements can also be an aggravating factor for arthritis. This can only be diagnosed accurately by whole-blood examination. For that reason red blood cells have to be included in the investigation, because the intracellular elements cannot be determined accurately in the blood serum. For that purpose red blood cells, the erythrocytes, have to be turned to ashes, and out of these the trace elements have to be determined.

Magnesium can also be detected more accurately by including the red blood cells into the test, because many elements are mostly located within the cells and not so much in the serum. Supplementation of the missing elements can take place, if the deficiencies have been determined accurately.

Chinese preparations for inflammatory joint problems will be listed at the end of this book as well as homeopathic remedies.

Asthma and related problems

Asthma was already mentioned with allergies, but it is expedient to again point out the essentials of that disease. There seems to be a genetic trait to asthma, it can be the consequence of allergies with inflammation of diverse kinds, which mostly take place in the respiratory tract. It starts in the windpipe (trachea) and goes down to the bronchi and bronchioles. It is mostly an inflammation of the mucus membranes of the trachea and the bronchi leading down into the smaller structures called bronchioles, and it is accompanied by a constriction of the underlying muscles as well.

Because of the inflammation the common treatment consists of cortisone, which counteracts the inflammation, and a beta-mimetic drug either as inhalation or in another form.

A relatively new drug is Montelucast, brandname Singulair®, which is a leukotriene antagonist.

Leukotrienes are inflammatory mediators that are mainly produced in leukocytes. They are usually accompanied by histamine and prostaglandins, which also initiate inflammation, especially in the course of an allergic process.

Montelucast helps to stop the wheezing, but as it does not act immediately, it should be taken for a longer time. As asthma is of allergic origin it may help to test for the allergens in order to be able to evade them. Sometimes testing turns out to be rather complicated, as the inhalable allergens in the environment are so numerous. Test sets do not contain all the possibilities that are present. So the patient has to observe the circumstances under which the allergy occurs.

Even food intolerances can lead to asthmatic symptoms without the possibility of a simple test. As there are no antibodies present, they are so-called pseudo-allergies, but the reaction can be the same as with real allergies.

Because the orthodox treatment with beta-mimetic drugs and cortisone has been known for a long time, we will not linger on that subject, but point out the alternatives.

In biological medicine we try the approach of cleansing with herbal substances, often accompanied by nosodes of inherited weaknesses like Tuberculinum, Psorinum or nosodes of pediatric diseases such as Varicella or Pertussis (whooping cough). They have to be given in higher potencies as well as nosodes of virus infections of various kinds such as Infuencinum and EBV.

Residues of vaccinations can turn out to be acting as toxins if too many vaccines had been given at the same time. At an early age a child's immune system may not be able to cope with a load of six or seven vaccines, all in one preparation.

In this case the corresponding nosodes could be tried as a treatment in order to take out the side effects that came along with that vaccination. That does not interfere with the protection against the respective illness gained by vaccination, only takes out the side effects for the immune system. In the treatment of children with asthma and eczema we saw many favourable changes with this therapeutic approach.

For cases of emergency caused by allergic shock or severe wheezing with asthma, cortisone should be kept at hand as an aerosole, but in most cases that remedy is disposable in the course of the treatment with homeopathy, as children usually respond very well.

Asthma and other allergies can change from one form of manifestation into another, for instance from eczema to asthma in a vicarious manner.

That phenomenon is not uncommon when symptoms are only suppressed and the causes are not thoroughly eliminated. Vicarious replacement (changing one for the other) can also happen in cases of desensitisation.

This regimen is applied to gain tolerance for an allergen such as pollen by injecting very small doses of the substance and then gradually increasing the amount.

But it can happen that only the allergy manifestation changes, not the allergic disposition. Instead of an allergy against certain pollen the patient could end up with food intolerances or allergies against other substances.

For adult asthmatic patients juice fasting turned out to act favourably, and certain vegetables and spices can also help, when added to the regimen. We would recommend garlic, onions or horse radish added to juices such as a green drink with cucumbers, celery and zucchini, or to red beet and carrot juice.

In cases of pollen allergies it makes sense for these people to eat honey with pollen therein, this seems to be a natural kind of desensitisation, as the pollen in this sort of honey can gradually get a person's immune system to accepting pollen as part of our natural environment.

There are quite a number of homeopathic remedies that can be used to help asthma patients, as for instance Spongia, Rumex, Kalium iodatum or Cuprum aceticum.

In Chinese Medicine they describe several forms of asthma, and it makes a great difference for the therapy if it is a wind-cold or a wind–hot form of asthma, or if there is a lot of mucus that has to be expelled. For the latter the citrus and Pinellia formula would be fitting in order to get rid of the phlegm. But first you have to find out what sort of asthma you are dealing with according to the 8 criteria, and by feeling the pulses and inspecting the tongue and the rest of the body after a thorough questioning.

When you have come to a diagnosis you can decide, which herbs are indicated or which acupuncture points can help to alleviate the symptoms.

As there are interactions between most organs, asthma can be caused by impairments of different organs and energetic systems.

Therapies can also differ considerably according to the cause of the disease. It can demand the Fritillaria and Ligusticum formula in one case, and in another the Ginseng and Astragalus formula, which will best be able to cope with the disease or at least help with the symptoms. Chinese herbs and formulas will be given later in detail.

The results of this form of therapy can be very rewarding if applied properly.

Baldness and hair loss

Baldness can have genetic roots as in androgenic baldness. Androgens, the male sex hormones, also play a certain role in women, as every human being produces androgens and estrogens, only the concentration of those hormones differs between men and women.

Anti-androgens, can be used for treatment, if the male sexual hormones play a role in baldness. This may be the case if severe hair loss or the following ailments occur: acne, seborrhoea or hirsutism, which means strong growth of hair on the body other than the head.

In that case youg women are concerned, they can replace the second hormone in birth control pills, the gestagen, which usually is derived from androgens, with the anti-androgen cyproterone acetate, which also acts as a gestagen. That way we get a remedy against androgenic hair loss.

Hair growth on the body is stimulated by androgens, but on the scalp they cause hair loss. Hair growth on the scalp on the other hand can be enhanced by taking Biotin, Zinc, silica as powder or certain homeopathic preparations of thallium. This makes sense when we remember the homoeopathic reverse action created by potentizing substances that in concentration act as toxins, as thallium does.

Foods rich in favourable substances are nuts, seeds and fresh vegetables, they are valuable, as they contain minerals, trace elements and enzymes. Vegetables counteract acidosis, because they are alkaline, which is not only favourable for hair growth but also for bone and joint metabolism.

Junk food and stress can also lead to hair loss, this is another reason to prefer fresh homemade meals, and not to rely on processed food out of the microwave oven or fast food as regular nutrition.

Juice fasting and detoxifying the body will have favourable results in the long run, using juices with onions or garlic for joint and hair problems, and herbal teas like Dandelion root or Gentian root that help to cleanse the liver.

It is a lot more complicated when the so-called alopecia areata is the reason for hair loss.

This is a localized form, mostly round in shape, where hair is disappearing with the tendency of bald spots gradually becoming larger. In this case an autoimmune disease is the underlying reason. In recent years it appears more frequently, especially in women. Stress seems to be a starting factor, but there is a strong genetic trait to that illness, as is the case in most autoimmune diseases.

We have seen certain improvements with autoimmune nosodes and detoxifying regimens. But in most cases it goes along with other manifestations of autoimmune diseases such as hypothyroidism. So the whole complex has to be taken care of, as it is not a localized phenomenon, but a generalized aberration of the immune system.

Homoeopathic treatment with thallium preparations in higher potency and Schuessler salts like calcium fluoratum or silica can be tried. Often nosodes of inherited weaknesses can be helpful, such as Medorrhinum and Luesinum, which in our experience often play a role in all kinds of autoimmune diseases.

In Chinese Medicine hair growth is seen in context with the hereditary energy and substance (Jing), which every being gets from his (her) parents. It is connected to the kidney, and it should very well be taken care of, because this inherited energy can be wasted too fast. This can happen if people are working too much or suffer from mental stress for longer periods.

All that diminishes also the Yin (the substance) and leads to a state of depletion, therefore the kidney energy and Jing should be replenished by taking herbal formulas, such as Rehmannia 6, which are helpful in building up substance and eliminating deficiencies.

Even massaging the scalp can be of advantage, as it improves the circulation in hair roots. Thus the accompanying constriction of little arteries can be counteracted, which often is brought about by stress.

B- vitamins as well as biotin and trace elements such as selenium can also help to improve hair growth.

Cancer development

As we move to the letter C, we have to take a close look at factors enhancing the development of cancer.

It is not amazing to see that cancer rates have increased as the consequences of pollution. There are toxins in air, water and food, some such as food preservatives, are being put there deliberately because everything has to be kept from decaying, and due to lack of time cannot be made freshly.

Others are residues such as insecticides, fungicides or nitrates out of mineral fertilizers. Genetically modified plants can also be hazardous, as nobody knows how they will affect living organisms in the long run.

But we pay a high price for our convenience, as the quality of our food is low, and we consume substances that can cause allergies or provoke degenerative diseases such as diabetes or cancer.

Carcinogenic substances can come from the outside, as is the case with food, water or air, or from the inside when they originate in our own intestines in the course of digestion.

We know that the intake of large quantities of red meat leads to a higher rate of colonic cancer because of toxic substances such as scatole, indole, putrescine or cadaverine being produced in the large bowel. Those metabolites have their origin in the slow or incomplete digestion of meat fibres in our bowel with consecutive rotting of proteins.

We also know that LDL cholesterol is increased through the consumption of animal fat and protein, not to mention chemical residues of antibiotics, sedatives and other detrimental substances, which have been found in meat.

They are used to enhance weight gain and prevent infections of animals in facilities for mass production of meat.

All those chemical residues will act in an unfavourable way on the cells of the inner layers of our digestive tract. That way cancer can develop through mutations in our DNA, which contains the genetic information for every cell.

In order to see what can happen we have to make a short excursion into genetics to come to an understanding what the DNA (deoxyribonucleic acid) consists of.

In most organisms, including humans, DNA is the hereditary material, laid down in chromosomes, which determines the structure and function of a body. Besides the DNA in the nucleus, there is a smaller portion of DNA in the cell organelles called mitochondria. The information is stored as a code made up of four nitrogen-containing bases. Two of them, the purine bases, have a double ring structure, (as shown in the picture), these are Adenine (A) and Guanine (G). Two of them, the pyrimidine bases, have a single ring structure, those are Cytosine (C) and Thymine (T).

Three billion bases constitute the human DNA, the sequence of which has been determined in 2000 by Craig Venter in the USA. The bases pair up by linking one double ring base (purine base) with one single ring base (pyrimidine base). That means, Adenine is always linked with Thymidine, and Cytosine is linked with Guanine.

Each base is attached to a sugar and a phosphate molecule, and together they form a nucleotide. Those nucleotides are arranged in long strands, and form a spiral that is called the double helix.

Every cell in an organism contains the same information in its chromosomes, that means with renewal of cells those

strands have to be replicated by making exact copies of the double helix.
At this point mistakes can happen, if conditions are unfavourable.

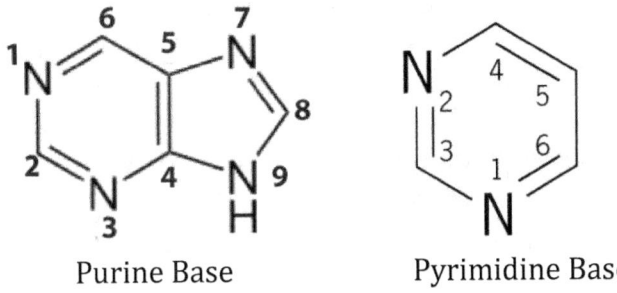

Purine Base   Pyrimidine Base

1

These can be toxic influences such as radiation, viruses or chemicals, thus mutations in that intricate system can be brought about.
If that happens, the cell is no longer the same, as base sequences can be altered, and translocation or breaking of chromosome parts can take place.
In some cases mutations are not life threatening, but it can as well be that new cells develop into cancer cells or other severe defects appear.
Only slight changes of the base sequences in the DNA can cause major disturbances leading to disastrous consequences. This is quite frequent under the influence of radiation, as we could witness after the Chernobyl disaster in 1986 when special forms of cancer became more frequent than they had been before, and often malformations in humans and animals could be seen.

All that refers to the nuclear DNA, but there is a second type called mitochondrial DNA, which is different from the nuclear one. It is transmitted exclusively in the maternal line, because the sperm in contrast to the ovum casts off all of the mitochondrial DNA in the course of its formation.

This special type can be of forensic importance, as in many old cases it may be still available when the nuclear DNA has already decayed. Then relatives in the maternal line have to be found in order to have a comparison with the DNA of the victim.

All DNA is susceptible to mutations, so we should be very careful in order to avoid toxins and radiation wherever we can, knowing that we are surrounded by plenty of hazardous substances anyway.

Though we have heard of the dangerous consequences of radioactivity that has been set free in nuclear testings and nuclear disasters like Chernobyl or Fukushima, we currently see that most people will have to live in the surrounding of their home country, as has been the case in Ukraine or Japan.

Radiation through x-rays or computer-tomography can also cause harm, as there is no absolutely innocuous radiation dose. Only the probability to cause some mutation in our DNA becomes higher with higher doses.

At least we should avoid adding other detrimental influences such as smoking, and should try to avoid exhaust fumes, which contain hundreds of toxic substances being potential carcinogens.

Therefore exercises should not take place in polluted air, and our food should be as fresh as possible and organically grown, especially if cancer or precancerosis is already present or runs in the family.

The reason is that a healthy body can eliminate cells, which have undergone mutation with the assistance of the cellular immune system. It consists of B and T-lymphocytes, which are subdivided into T-suppressor and T-helper cells, the latter being further divided into natural killer cells and cytotoxic T-cells.

They are very important for the detection and elimination of cell aberrations, as they cause cells with mutations to commit suicide, which is called apoptosis. This will be further explained later in this chapter. Those processes take place hundreds of times during our lifetime, so that potentially dangerous cells in most cases can be detected and destroyed in a healthy organism.

To keep the cellular immune system in good shape it is essential to have an intact intestinal flora.

For that reason we try to avoid toxic and rotting substances in our bowel, and take an effort to get the life sustaining substances we mentioned earlier in this book, such as secondary plant substance, which act as antioxidants.

Besides eating fresh and unprocessed food, also juices of certain vegetables such as carrots and red beets or zucchini and cucumbers together with celery, garlic and onions can help to keep the body in a healthy balance.

Minerals and trace elements together with B-vitamins and kelp powder or tablets are of advantage. Sour milk products are helpful for the intestinal flora, especially when they contain live cultures of acidophilus bacteria.

Herbs to cleanse the liver are recommended in anyway.

In many European countries preparations of mistletoe are used to enhance the immune system and injections of thymus preparations are also available for use after cancer surgery.

In order to monitor cancer patients properly we use to have a thorough examination not only of the normal blood count, but also of the cellular immune profile. This is important, as it shows the sub groups of T-lymphocytes such as natural killer cells and cytotoxic T-cells.

They attack the cells, which have undergone mutation into malignant cells by secreting lymphokines, which typically are produced by T-lymphocytes. Those lymphokines lead to an immune system response between cells, and they can attract other immune cells to an infected site. Besides that they help B-cells producing antibodies and can cause apoptosis in cells, which have undergone mutation. Thus these cells will commit suicide and be eliminated.

Therefore the cellular immune response should be carefully monitored, as it is essential in fighting cancer. Mostly the cellular immune system is impaired after the orthodox cancer treatment with radiation and/or chemotherapy after surgery. The recovery of the cellular immune system is much faster with the help of thymus and mistletoe preparations and the rebuilding of a healthy bowel flora.

As already mentioned there are also viruses, which can cause cervical cancer, such as the dangerous subtypes 16 and 18 of the Human Papilloma Virus. The now existing vaccination against those two types can be recommended for girls after puberty, as long as they had no contact with those viruses, but it does not contain all the dangerous types and has to be repeated after a few years, as the immunity does not last very long.

The Epstein Barr Virus can also lead to a type of cancer, if people come in connection with a substance called phorbol ester. That substance is contained in the sap of certain plants, which can promote the development of a special kind of lymphoma. This is not uncommon in Africa after contact with a plant called Croton tiglium, which contains those phorbol esters.

They seem to interact with membranes of cells making them more permeable for viruses. The resulting Burkitt lymphoma is a fast growing Non Hodgkin lymphoma, with a high degree of malignancy. Sporadic cases of that lymphoma have also been reported in other countries such a China.

Lymphomas take place in the core of the immune system and consist of different sorts of T- or B-lymphocytes. There exists a whole system of classification for these tumours.

Normal B-cell lymphocytes are the source of the so-called humoral immune system. They transform into plasma cells and produce immune globulins of different types called alpha, beta and gamma globulins. The gamma type is divided into several subgroups, such as the IG_E, which is elevated in case of allergies.

The T-or thymus lymphocytes are divided into T-helper and T-suppressor cells, the percentage of both indicates what state the immune system is in. When the helper part drops too low this is a sign of a depressed immune system. We have seen that happen in cases of severe HIV infection, even before AIDS was manifested.

Natural killer and cytotoxic T-cells are responsible for the system called the cellular immune response. This means the immune cells act directly on other cells with the help of lymphokines, but without the interception of immune globulines.

The Chinese approach to these problems is quite different, as it tries to regulate deficiencies and stagnations in energy flow. Weak organs get help to detoxify and rebuild energy and substance. In the end that also builds up a better

153

immune defence against cells that have changed and been led astray to kill its own organism.

This approach makes sense, because cancer should not be considered a local problem that can be solved by cutting out the malignant cells in a certain organ, but with a holistic approach the whole organism is considered sick and should be treated accordingly by cleansing all the important organs and the lymph system.

Cardiologic problems

Problems connected to the heart comprise a wide variety of symptoms and manifestations. They can be in connection with inflammation of the valves that connect the atria and ventricles or the ventricles with the lungs and the aorta. The mitral valve seems to be the most vulnerable, as even in young individuals stenosis (narrowing) or insufficiency of that valve occur as a consequence of inflammation.

This inflammation mostly takes place in the tonsils and pharynx and can become chronic. Therefore it should be taken care of before damage has happened to valves or myocardium (heart muscle).

With older people we get more and more problems with the aortic valve that connects the left ventricle to the whole body circulation via the aorta. Arrhythmias and tachycardia can be the consequence of inflammation, valvular disease or coronary problems. Malnutrition of the heart muscle ensues mostly from problems with blood circulation due to coronary artery disease. When one or more coronary arteries are clogged the consequence is a heart attack (infarction), because the hard working heart muscle no longer gets sufficient blood supply.

154

We will have to consider how the heart itself can be strengthened after an infarction in order to prevent another one. If the circulation is impaired by atherosclerosis, we will have to think about remedies to alleviate the ailments.

The orthodox therapy with diuretics, beta-blockers, ACE inhibitors and nitrates is well known, so we will not have to linger on that topic.

There are several homeopathic remedies that can be used to strengthen the heart muscle. They have to be selected according to the special symptoms and modalities.

Valuable remedies for impaired circulation can be the snake poisons Naja tripudians (cobra) and Lachesis muta (bushmaster) and a number of other snake poisons such as Crotalus horridus (rattle snake), they should not be used in a low potency, but from D or C12 upward, as explained in the chapter on homeopathy.

Besides that, numerous plants can enhance the action of the heart as for instance convallaria maialis (lily of the valley), Galanthus nivalis (snowdrop), Adonis, Crataegus and many more.

The Chinese medical system aims at restoring the energy situation of the heart and helping to get rid of an overload of fluid, which has become a burden for the actions of the heart. For that purpose quite a number of herbs or specific formulas are available.

Chronic inflammation of the bowel

Chronic bowel problems, which can be caused by inflammatory processes such as Crohn's disease, will be our next topic.

Crohn's disease can take place in any part of the intestinal system, but the predominant location is the terminal small bowel, the ileum. That is why it is also called Ileitis terminalis.

But it can as well affect the colon and make the discernment from colitis quite difficult. It can spread deep in the layers of the intestinal mucus membranes (tunica mucosa). There it can cause strictures, ulcerations and even fistula, between different bowel parts or bowel and bladder.

There seem to be genetic and immunological causes and the response to bacteria in the intestinal mucosa is impaired.

Orthodox therapy consists of the suppression of the immune system with substances such as cortisone, azathioprine, mercaptopurine, sulfasalazine or infiximab (Remicade®). The latter is a tumour necrosis factor inhibitor, which is also used for other autoimmune diseases.

As we have explained that class of remedies already in the chapter on arthritis, we won't have to go into details again. With this kind of therapy the immunological response to antigens is modified and the inflammation is held down. People with a history of cancer, though, should not take tumour necrosis factor inhibitors, which are monoclonal antibodies, because the immune system will be suppressed that way. as a consequence a relapse of the illness could happen more easily or other problems may arise.

Mostly cortisone is used as first therapeutic approach together with Sulfasalazine or Mesalazine, drugs which are also used for the treatment of ulcerative colitis.
But frequently those substances are not well tolerated.

Therefore we tried another regime with cleansing of the bowel and building up of a new flora. Besides that liver therapy with cleansing herbs and changing of lifestyle is advisable. Omitting sugar and simple carbohydrates while substituting minerals and trace elements such as zinc and selenium is expedient. The illness cannot be cured, but it can be kept stable for certain periods, if patients decide to stick to their diet and change their lifestyle, where alcohol and smoking have no place.
 Another inflammatory disease is ulcerative colitis, which is situated in the lower part of the bowel, the colon and rectum. But it does not cause fistulas as Crohn's does, but is limited to the mucosa. Nevertheless it can be accompanied by severe diarrhoea with blood and parts of the mucosa appearing with the stool.
The orthodox treatment consists mostly of cortisone and mesalazine, the latter is given in different ways of application, from oral tablets to enemas and locally applied foam. There can be remissions, but mostly relapses follow from time to time. In recent years tumour necrosis factor inhibitors have also been tried for this disease.
With the biological approach to colitis we can often see a different outcome when patients first treat the diarrhoea with psyllium seed, and then try to omit gluten in their diet. That means to live for a certain time without any normal bread. If all grain products are omitted, it is easier to cope with the intestinal inflammation and to stop the diarrhoea.

In case gluten problems have been suspected, it seems logical to replace normal bread by the gluten-free variety, or replace bread with millet and buckwheat as they are well tolerated, as well as rice and corn (maize) products.

Sour milk products are helpful to restore the bowel flora, if they contain live cultures of acidophilus bacteria.

The most common result of bowel problems is excessive gas formation, which stems in almost all cases from alterations of the bowel flora. This mostly happens after application of antibiotics or treatment with chemotherapy.

Building up a new bowel flora is the main target, and there are several good preparations on the market with lactobacillus acidophilus or bifidus cultures or even a modified Escherichia coli preparation (Mutaflor®).

A diet with less meat and more protein from nuts and seeds and more vegetables together with less sugar and white meal products is also of advantage.

The energetic approach of Chinese medicine with herbs plus acupuncture/acupressure could as well influence the disease in a favourable way. In that case herbal formula for the liver function will have to be included.

The homeopathic therapy with salmonella or colitis nosodes accompanied by cleansing herbs showed good results, if accompanied by remedies that fit the constitution of the patient.

The next important topic will be diabetes mellitus, which not only shows elevated blood sugar, but also metabolic disturbances in connection with blood lipids and uric acid.

There are two main types of diabetes, which show major differences concerning their etiology and their treatment.

158

Diabetes

Type1 diabetes is a disease where the beta cells in the islets of Langerhans in the pancreas do not produce insulin, because they suffered or were destroyed in an autoimmune process. This form can be found in children as well as in adults and has to be treated with insulin. Fortunately Insulin had been found by Banting and Best in 1921, and was later made available. It was detected in the pancreas of dogs, and insulin of animal source was used for a long time, especially the porcine type and also the bovine type.

But as the human insulin is different from the animal insulin in the sequence of amino acids, it was a great progress when pharmaceutical companies started producing human insulin in 1975. This is mostly done with the help of bacteria (Escherichia coli) with the aid of gene transfer into these organisms.

Contrary to the first type, where patients are mostly slender, the type2 diabetes is found in obese patients. Their tissues are insensitive to insulin because the whole metabolism is out of balance.

This form can, at least in the beginning, be treated with tablets such as Metformin, according to orthodox medicine.

As the rapid increase of diabetic patients during the last 30 years suggests, it has to do with our unhealthy western lifestyle with overeating and lack of exercise. So the first thing to do for overweight type 2 diabetic patients is to change eating habits and start on more exercise.

Our recommendation goes to less animal protein, fat and sugar and to more fresh food like fruit and vegetables together with complex carbohydrates.

That way weight can be lost and less medication will be necessary.

Only if that goal cannot be reached, Metformin can be tried.

Our biologic approach would go farther and start with herbal support, with plants such as Coccinia cardifolia, Hintonia latiflora, bitter melon juice, and cinnamon powder, if not more than 5 grams per day were ingested. These herbs have no side effects when applied in the recommended doses.

There are also homeopathic remedies such as Syzygium jambolanum to enhance the insulin production. Herbs like Maca or cats' claw can be used for further metabolic support.

In Mexico the indigenous population used to eat cactus pads, which are made out of cactus leaves to treat diabetes, and they seem to have had some success with that. Our patients usually received supplements of vitamins B and E and the trace elements chromium, selenium and zinc. Chromium is specifically protective for diabetic patients.

It cannot be expected that type1 diabetes can be cured, but we can get good results if overweight persons with type 2 diabetes apply those recommendations. Often they will be able to stop their tablet intake with the suggested therapy.

In cases of type 2 diabetes also fasting can be recommended and later a diet with a great portion of fibres in it. That way we create a different blood sugar curve. Complex carbohydrates imbedded in lots of fibre cause the sugar curve after meals to stay in an acceptable range, and it is kept steadier for a longer interval.

If the diabetic patient also suffers from osteoarthritis, which impedes normal sportive activities, swimming or using a home trainer bike can help with the weight loss program.

We see good results with that regimen, and that way consequences of diabetes such as atherosclerosis can be kept at bay. Coronary heart disease, strokes or loss of an extremity because of impaired circulation, nephropathy or eye problems like diabetic retinopathy will be less frequent when blood sugar levels are kept steadier.

Gout as a result of elevated uric acid

Another metabolical illness is gout, as it is caused by the deposition of uric acid in joints and tissues. The reasons for elevated uric acid levels can be either faulty nutrition or the inability of the kidneys to excrete that substance in a proper way.

Purine bases (s. picture on page 149) are the source of uric acid. There are the two nitrogen bases with the structure of a purine double ring structure, Adenine and Guanine, which are part of DNA and of RNA.

The Crick Watson model of DNA shows in an impressive way the structure of the double helix. It is built up of nucleotides containing bases, sugar molecules and phosphoric acid. But besides the DNA, also RNA (ribonucleic acid) is essential.

As messenger RNA it transfers the information for the building of proteins from the DNA into the cytoplasma. different sugars, ribose and deoxyribose, discern the two.

In contrast to DNA, the RNA contains a different base instead of thymine, and that is uracil.

In humans and mammals the genetic code is composed of DNA, but RNA plays an important role in the protein synthesis. This happens through transcription and translation from the base sequence of the DNA.

161

Transcription means the information is transferred to the RNA by the coupling of complementary bases between RNA and DNA. Translation is the changing into proteins by using three bases as code for one amino acid, as for instance the base sequence CAU, which stands for the amino acid valin.

Every amino acid has a specific code, so that all sorts of proteins can be built up that way.

In contrast to DNA the RNA does not form a double-helix, but is mono-stranded.

All cell material containing purine bases is responsible for the formation of uric acid, and as even plants contain it, but to a lesser degree, they can also contribute. Nevertheless, the main source are tissues of animals, for instance liver and other organs. But also muscle tissue contains cell nuclei, and therefore is a source of uric acid.

So our food should not have an overload of organ meat, especially when a genetic trait exists causing the problem of slow excretion of uric acid in our kidneys. In that case the nutrition should be adjusted to that condition and the intake of cell material be kept low. Otherwise patients will have to take tablets that keep the uric acid level down, as does the substance allopurinol. That is a synthetic remedy, which interferes with the building of uric acid, as the molecule is similar. It is not always well tolerated, as hypersensitivity reactions can appear. Besides that it is toxic for the liver and therefore dangerous.

We would rather recommend cutting down on the intake of proteins containing cells, i.e. meat products, certain sorts of fish, which also contain a heavy load of purines like mackerel, herring and sardines. Problems can also arise with

162

legumes like peas, beans and lentils, as they are sources for purines, but to a lesser extent.

Proteins that contain no cells such as milk products cannot form uric acid. But not all sorts of protein containing cows' milk are well tolerated by sensitive or allergic patients, so it is best to use goats' milk.

In any case, some support has to be given for the kidneys, as they have to excrete the uric acid. This can be done with herbal teas like Juniper, Solidago or Equisetum (horsetail). Enough liquid is also important, so the kidneys can excrete the waste products more easily. It can happen that the uric acid levels go up during a fast, because old cell material is cleared out, but that is usually only transitory and never leads to complications, if enough liquid is offered for the cleansing process.

Hypertension as a risk factor

Another important topic we will have to deal with is hypertension or high blood pressure.

The reasons for high blood pressure can be manifold, because it is a reaction of the body to different underlying pathological conditions and stress.

In many cases we have found emotional disturbances to be the reason. It should be the goal to eliminate the underlying causes before starting a therapy with diuretics or other substances for blood pressure such as beta-blockers or ACE inhibitors.

Mostly the renal function is also slightly impaired, though it can be hard to detect. The parameters for the function of the kidneys, such as creatinine, only show major impairments. That is understandable, as the kidneys have plenty of reserve capacity, before parameters like creatinine or urea show any pathological findings. You can even donate one of your kidneys and still have normal values and a satisfactory function.

When the hormonal balance is altered, high blood pressure can appear for the first time. We had patients where exactly that happened during pregnancy, but no major impairments as for liver or kidney function were to be found in laboratory tests.

In one case, where the hypertension persisted after the birth of the baby, the mother was treated with synthetic medications for a number of years. We were not content with the outcome and started a therapy with homoeopathic remedies and nosodes. The result was that within a few weeks the blood pressure was gradually coming down, though the high pressure had been there for six years. Nevertheless did we continue the therapy with renal nosodes and homoeopathic preparations plus Chinese and western herbal medicine. We gradually got the blood pressure back to normal, and it stayed normal in the end without any medication.

As hormones play an important role in the maintenance of blood pressure, hormonal disturbances can also be significant in connection with phaeochromocytoma. This is an adenoma of the adrenal medulla producing epinephrine, which can be the reason for hypertension. The stress hormone epinephrine (adrenaline) among other things pushes up the blood pressure.

In case of an emergency epinephrine can be necessary to prepare for fight or flight, but the constant elevation poses a risk of its own. The same applies to hyperthyroidism, which can also cause high blood pressure. The hormone thyroxin, besides creating high blood pressure enhances our alertness and metabolism, and it also causes tachycardia, heart arrhythmia and insomnia.

Cushing's syndrome, where cortisole is too high, shows elevated blood sugar and inadequate actions of our immune system besides being able to cause high blood pressure. The growth of new fibrous tissue is also impeded, as well as the building of new bone structure.

Hypertension is a risk factor for stroke, myocardial infarction and congestive heart failure, as the heart has to do heavy work to create that high pressure. Inflammation and degenerative changes in the walls of our arteries can play a major role in creating high blood pressure, especially if it leads to stenosis (narrowing) in the renal arteries. Even overweight as a risk factor can end up causing hypertension, as many hormones are produced in fat tissue. Important

165

ones are oestrogens and leptin, which is an appetite suppressor. Hormone production mostly takes place in fat cells of the abdomen.

Smoking has been found to be detrimental, as the toxic substances in tobacco smoke cause spasms that can obstruct already impaired arteries in a bad way.

The overall rate of hypertension worldwide is about 20%, but there are great differences. When we consider India with 3 to 5 % compared to countries like the United States or Europe with 30%, we wonder what may be the reason. Plenty of salt, which is traditionally used in those countries, and the western diet with consecutive overweight seem to contribute to that difference.

It is plausible that a change in lifestyle has to be the first thing to be done. The most important steps to take are cutting down on salt, reducing the fat intake, and consuming less meat.

Then a cleansing program with herbs for the liver and kidneys, together with a fast could further help to get out of that vicious cycle. More exercise can be helpful, as it tends to reduce weight and is beneficial for our metabolism.

Hypertension in view of Chinese medicine can have many different reasons, therefore we will give a few examples of what that means concerning this disease.

Hypertension caused by so-called liver fire conditions, mostly as a consequence of severe mental or emotional problems, includes dizziness, headache, irritability, restlessness or nightmares. It should be treated with liver formulas soothing that condition and coping with the emotional problems.

Hypertension caused by deficient kidney yin includes symptoms such as lower back pain, tinnitus, palpitations, shortness of breath and so on, and it can be treated with formulas such as Rehmannia 6, which build up the yin of the kidneys.

Hypertension by blood deficiency shows pale skin and tongue, palpitations, insomnia and poor appetite, and it can be treated by blood building formulas such as Ginseng 8.

The overall results can see with all the mentioned regimens were good, if patients decided to stick to it for a certain length of time, as the results cannot be obtained in a few days.

Liver problems

Our next topic are diseases of the liver, and they comprise quite a number of things from chronic hepatitis after an acute infection with a virus out of the hepatitis family to all sorts of reactions to toxic substances.

There are several forms of hepatitis, i.e. the inflammation of the liver, either by viruses, bacteria or through toxicity of substances in our environment. A special form is autoimmune hepatitis, this is the illness, which is least understood.

The A- type hepatitis is the one with the best prognosis, because it rarely becomes chronic. It is mostly transmitted oral-faecally, that means it can be transmitted from contaminated fingers to food, and thus another person may be infected. In developing countries this takes place in early childhood, and it leaves people with lifelong immunity. In western countries it occurs much later, if at all, as the standard of hygiene is usually higher. Most infected children have but slight symptoms, accompanying the illness, and are left with a lifelong immunity.

In 1991 a vaccination against this type of hepatitis was developed that gives a relatively good immunity but not a lifelong one, so it may prove necessary to repeat the procedure after ten or so years.

The B-type hepatitis on the other hand poses more of a problem, since it tends to become chronic in 10 to 20 percent. This can lead to liver cirrhosis, and end up as liver cell carcinoma.

Vaccination is available, which yields a good protection and is given routinely in developed countries. It should best be applied around the age of puberty, because then the risk of contracting that virus goes up considerably.

As a consequence of the vaccination, infection rates in those countries have become less. Still one third of the world's population has had contact with the virus, and there are numerous carriers who harbour the virus for a long time and transmit it to other people. That takes place mostly by body fluids or contact with blood. So it can be a bad surprise after sex tourism to come home with B-type hepatitis.

The gravest problems are created by the C-type hepatitis, because chronic infection can lead to scarification of the liver. This disease is mostly contracted by intra-venous drug use or by blood transfusion. Also inadequately sterilised surgical equipment or tattooing can be the cause. It tends to become chronic in about 80% of the cases, especially if co-infection with B-type hepatitis or HIV exists. It can lead to liver cirrhosis with the risk of bleeding from oesophageal or gastric varicose veins. It has become the most frequent reason for liver transplants, and it can end up as liver cell carcinoma.

Transmission from mother to infant is possible during pregnancy or delivery, but it only happens in about 10% of cases. Sexual transmission can occur, but is not that frequent as with the B-type hepatitis.

An estimated 200 million people in the world suffer from chronic C-type hepatitis, and there is no vaccine available yet.

For the C-type hepatitis new therapeutic approaches have been devised during the past years with peginterferon and ribavirin, with possible addition of boceprevir or telaprevir. Ribavirin is a prodrug, which is metabolized into a molecule that resembles purine RNA nucleotides. Thus the viral replication is hindered, as this faulty nucleotide is blocking the replication of the virus, which is an RNA virus.

Ribavirin can cause haemolytic anaemia and is a teratogen, which means a potential hazard for the formation of cancer. The antiviral agents boceprevir and telaprevir can shorten the time for therapy and increase the percentage of cures from that virus. But they have considerable side effects too, mostly on the blood building system causing anaemia.

Still on the whole the untreated hepatitis C poses the greater risk.

There are other viruses that can cause hepatitis, for instance the EBV, Lassa, Ebula or the Marburg virus, as well as Dengue, Chikungunya and Yellow fever. Though a possibility for vaccination against Yellow fever exists, there have been quite a number of complications as a consequence. They appeared mostly as flu-like with fever and muscle pain, headache or allergic symptoms with a rash and even neurologic ailments.

For the other viruses there are no vaccines available, Lassa and Ebula have a high mortality rate, as we have seen in several cases of West Africa.

There have been outbreaks of Dengue in a number of countries in recent years, mostly in South America and South-east Asia.

The Chicungunya virus led to a severe outbreak on the isle of Réunion in 2006, but it had been first found in Tansania in 1953. Dengue and Chikungunia are transmitted by the same mosquito, namely Aedes Aegypti, but not exclusively.

Bacteria can also lead to a liver inflammation caused by agents such as Listeria or Leptospira . Listeria is one of the most virulent food-borne pathogens, it is sometimes found in soft cheese, and 20% to 30% of clinical infections result in death. Newborn babies can contract it from their mothers in the course of birth.

Leptospira bacteria can be found throughout the world, they can be transmitted from animals such as rats and cause Weil's disease of the liver.

Parasites such as Echinococcus (the so-called fox tapeworm) and protozoa such as Trypanosoma Cruci in South America or Leishmania Donovani in Africa can also cause hepatitis.

Then there is the mostly cryptic form, namely autoimmune hepatitis, which can be the consequence of certain diseases, toxins and drugs. In that case no causing agent can be found, and therefore it is treated by immune suppression, which in itself brings about many side effects.

Finally we will give a few examples to show which substances in the form of drugs or toxins can become a hazard for the liver function, as that organ may have difficulties to detoxify the synthetic substance or the natural poison.

1.   Amiodarone is a drug used against cardiac arrhythmias.
2.   Halothane is a gas for anaesthesia, replacing formerly used ether and chloroform, which are now obsolete.

3. Ibuprofen and Indometazine are painkillers and antirheumatics.

4. Hormonal contraception can contain various synthetic gestagens , which are derived from androgens, besides that the oestrogen ethinyl-oestradiol is contained in every combined contraceptive pill. Pure gestagens have to be deposited as an injection or implanted under the skin.

5. Ketoconazol is an antifungal, taken as tablets it can cause elevated liver enzymes.

6. Loratadine is an antihistamine against allergies like hay fever.

7. Methotrexate is an immune suppressive drug.

8. Paracetamol, also called acetaminophen is a painkiller and antipyretic (against fever), which can cause depression of the bone marrow apart from being liver toxic.

9. Phenytoin and valproic acid are antiepileptic drugs.

10. Zitovudine is used against the HI virus to prevent AIDS.

11. Haemochromatosis is a hereditary illness, where too much iron is deposited in vital organs, this can cause hepatitis and pancreatitis.

12. Morbus Wilson is due to copper accumulation in the body.

13. Amatoxin containing mushrooms are so toxic that 1 mg can kill a person, especially one mushroom is dangerous, and that is the so called death cap (Amanita phalloides), there is just one remedy against this toxin, which is an injectible concentrate out of the milk thistle (carduus marianus), produced by the German Madaus company.

14. Well known is the alcoholic hepatitis, and less known the hepatitis due to eclampsia during pregnancy, a

severe form of that is the so-called HELLP syndrome, the abbreviation stands for high blood pressure, elevated liver enzymes and low platelet count.

Those are only a few toxic agents out of a greater number, which have been mentioned here, as we only wanted to show how manifold the reasons for liver inflammations can be.
The aim of homoeopathic and other natural treatments on the other hand is to help the body overcome hepatitis of any type, so it will not become chronic and drift into cirrhosis. For that purpose the therapy should consist of several steps.

Liver cleansing of all the toxins from the environment should be the first step, and should start with heavy metals. We mentioned various methods, such as chelating therapy with the agents DMPS or DMSA. An alternative for less severe cases can be the Chlorella algae therapy.
The detoxification of residues from insecticides, herbicides and fungicides can be tried with homeopathy, as Drs R. Voll and C. Hagen had suggested by using high potencies of the same substance.

The therapy with herbal teas such as milk thistle, Gentian or Chinese herbal formulas can be applied after fasting.
Changing the entire diet to less fat, less sugar and more fresh food such as salads can also be recommended.
For people who had suffered from hepatitis there are several different nosodes available for treatment to keep the liver from developing cirrhosis, homeopathic organ preparations can be added.
Trying to lose excess weight by more exercise in fresh, unpolluted air is indispensible.

The portion of food with a low respiratory quotient, such as saturated fats, should be cut down, as they use too much oxygen in the course of digestion.

Many toxins, which have been stored in the liver, can be excreted via bile, which is produced in the liver. It is stored in our gall bladder, and when it becomes necessary for the process of digestion, it is excreted in our small bowel, where it is meant to emulsify the fats, as only very small fat droplets can be easily digested.

Excretion of toxins can be accomplished with herbs, which enhance the flux of bile, such as curcuma or chelidonium (celandine).

The liver is also very important from the standpoint of Chinese medicine, as it is the organ that dominates the flow of energies in the whole system, and it also rules the emotions.

It is called liver Qi- stagnation, when the energy does not flow properly. Then it moves upward creating migraine or headache, instead of ruling the digestive processes between stomach and spleen.

In severe cases it is called liver fire, which is mostly caused by violent emotions. This can also lead to headaches or migraine, which can be treated with acupuncture. It may later be followed by Chinese herbal formulas to restore the proper flow of the liver energy (the liver Qi).

Certain points can be used as acupuncture or acupressure points, especially on the gall bladder meridian in the head region, but also on the liver-, stomach-or bladder-meridian.

If given proper help the liver has some capacity to regenerate. We can see that from the fact that even with a small part of a liver transplanted, that organ can grow bigger and regain an appropriate function.

Lung problems

As the lungs are in close connection to the heart function, many diseases such as congestive heart failure will have an impact on the lungs. If the heart's action is insufficient, transport of blood from the lungs into the body circulation will suffer. As a consequence fluid will gather in the lungs and make proper breathing more and more difficult. In the end the whole circulation may break down.

As the lungs are the organ with the most immediate outside connection, all the toxins, present in the air we breathe, get into our lungs straight away, and from here into the blood stream.

That is why the inhalation of toxins is the most dangerous way to get into contact with them, as the penetration of the alveolar walls of the lung into the blood stream happens faster and more thoroughly than by any other way.

Therefore exercising in clean air with proper breathing is essential, as we need plenty of oxygen to create our own energy, in the form of ATP, in the electron transport chain.

The close connection with the outside world also brings us in close connection with allergens like pollen or toxic gases, as well as viruses or bacteria. These may be an influenza virus or the tuberculosis bacterium, which can be distributed by little droplets when a sick person is coughing.

All the different viruses like the avian flu or swine flu virus are prone to rapid mutations, and we get new influenza types almost every year. So it is almost impossible to build up permanent immunity against these attackers.

With tuberculosis it is different, but not better, as we have seen a development, where more and more multi-drug-resistant mycobacteria (the agent that causes tuberculosis) have emerged.

This means they do not respond to the tuberculostatica INH and Rifampicin, two of the most common remedies for this disease. Especially in Africa and parts of the former Soviet Union, this became a great problem, but also other countries are confronted with that situation. High doses of vitamin C seem helpful to overcome the resistance.

Considering all those facts we have good reasons to strengthen our immune system. This can be done with Chinese herbs, proper nutrition and detoxifying procedures like fasting or excretion of toxic metals. Residues of herbicides and other toxic substances of our environment can be excreted with the help of homeopathic substances as already described.

As we stated in the asthma chapter, there are quite a number of approaches to lung problems with Chinese medicine, which can be a good alternative to the orthodox treatment. A list of important Chinese herbs and a few formulas will be given at the end of this book.

Menstrual imbalances and other gynaecological problems

Menstrual imbalances will keep us occupied in this chapter, and we will try to look at those impairments from different angles. We will start with the view from the standpoint of Chinese medicine where everything depends on the proper flow of the energy called Qi.

There are several pathological patterns that can happen in the menstrual cycle. We will begin with the menstrual flow, which can be too strong or too weak as a consequence of imbalance in the flow of Qi.

Poor menstrual flow due to deficient liver and kidney energy can be accompanied by more symptoms like weak lower back, dizziness, night sweats, ringing in the ears, hot and dry tongue and mouth, and hot palms and soles. A good remedy for that would be the Rehmannia 6 formula, which will be presented in detail in the chapter on formulas.

Other reasons for menstrual problems can be deficient Qi and blood with paleness of the skin and tongue.

The Ginseng and Longan formula could be used as a remedy for that condition.

If blood stasis and Qi stagnation are the reason, we will see that the patient has a bluish dark tongue. He will also have a feeling of fullness in chest and abdomen with depression or irritability. Tang Gui 4, containing Angelica sinensis, could be used as a remedy in this case. When accompanied by pain or cramps, Corydalis (lark spur) may be added to that formula.

There could be many more combination of stagnation or deficiency, we only wanted to show with a few examples, how sophisticated the approach in Chinese medicine is, because the reasons for diseases can vary on a broad scale.

In treating similar conditions with homeopathy we have to look at the symptoms very closely, and find out as much as we can about the modalities, which means when, and under what conditions the problems with menstruation occur. We have to consider time of day or night, localisation of pain and last not least the mental state a person is in, when suffering from those ailments.

Then we can carefully select our remedy, which should fit that condition and the constitution of the patient.

For cramping pains we could choose Cuprum aceticum, and for bleeding that is too strong Viburnum opulus. The constitution of a patient is very important, as by choosing a constitutional remedy, which fits most of her characteristic traits, we create a foundation for therapy.

Accompanying mental stress, being responsible for many ailments in connection with the female monthly cycle, should be treated first. Ignatia or Lilium tigrinum can be of some help in that connection, if the remedy pictures fit for the patient.

This is another very individual way to treat patients, and it takes plenty of time and knowledge to select the correct remedies. This can be done with the help of a repertory or a materia medica, as for instance the famous "Boericke" where many symptoms are described in an accurate way, and still the book is small enough to fit into most pockets. Online repertories are also available, as well as books in several volumes, for instance the" Clark" in three volumes.

The orthodox therapy for gynecological problems is quite different, as it merely treats the symptoms the patients tell us. In cases of disturbances in the menstrual cycle, mostly hormones are given as a prescription under the premise that there may be a deficiency.

Gestagens are first choice, as they rule the second half of the cycle. The natural one is progesterone, but there are quite a number of synthetic gestagens in use. Levonorgestrel is one of those, it is often contained in birth control pills or gestagen-loaded intra-uterine coils. Also a combined substitution of estrogens and gestagens is often tried to restore the cycle, and the outcome shows, if this therapy was successful.

So in the end it is more an approach of trial and error than looking for the underlying reasons of illnesses.

But of course, it should never be forgotten that some conditions like bleedings, especially in the early or late menopause, may be a sign of uterine corpus cancer or precancerosis. Then an ultrasound check should be done, and the conditon can be diagnosed further by curettage or hysteroscopy.

The annual Pap smear for the diagnosis of cervical alterations such as dysplasia, which can occur at an earlier age, is quite a different procedure, as the reasons and the location of the cell alterations are quite different. We discussed that before in connection with Human Papilloma Virus, which is largely responsible for that disease.

Cancer of the uterine corpus mostly starts around the age of menopause or shortly before, when hormonal imbalances are frequent, but it can also be manifested later.

Ovarian cancer on the other hand can be diagnosed best by ultrasound, but the primary tumour may be quite small and can be easily overlooked. Often this tumour has already spread metastases when it is found.

Multiple Sclerosis

Now we will deal with a disease, which incapacitates patients who are confronted with it to a large extent, because it attacks the nervous system. We are talking of encephalomyelitis disseminata, also called multiple sclerosis. It affects the brain and the spinal cord, namely the fatty myelin sheaths surrounding the axons. Those are long projections or nerve fibres, which have to conduct electrical impulses away from the nerve cell, thus transmitting information and connecting cells with one another. Many parts of the body can be disturbed that way by loss of sensitivity, tingling or pricking sensations, numbness or muscle spasms. Eye sensations due to optic neuritis are quite frequent, as well as difficulties with coordination and balance. Many inner organs such as bladder, bowels or gullet may be impaired in their function too.

It is wellknown that an autoimmune process causes the attack on myelin sheaths, but the reasons for that process are discussed controversially.

Frequent virus infections that were not taken proper care of, and that had left residues of toxins in the body, can be a reason. Toxic substances from within or without seem to play a role as well as a genetic disposition. The disease is more frequent in countries with a colder climate, and there is a female preponderance.

With new therapies the underlying autoimmune process can be slowed down or stopped for a certain time, but that is not a cure in the literal sense.

Nevertheless the beta- interferon therapy has been a great improvement compared to the former attempts to suppress the immune system. If that is not tolerated well, the alternative could be Natalizumab, which is a monoclonal antibody. This substance can also be used for other autoimmune diseases, as we already mentioned in the chapter on arthritis.

Another alternative can be Copaxone® (Glatiramer-acetate), a synthetic immune modulator, developed in Israel. It can be given, if the interferon therapy leads to complications and has to be stopped.

This should not be the only way of treatment, but there could also be an attempt to detoxify the organism and help with proper nutrition. In our experience fresh organically grown food does those patients good. A high portion of raw vegetables together with cold pressed, unprocessed oil in salads has turned out to be quite helpful to maintain or regain strength and keep the disease from getting worse. Lactic acid fermented vegetables like sauerkraut, cucumbers or others prepared in the same way, are much better than the pickled variety containing acetic acid.

Coffee and strong black tea as well as sugar should be omitted, and canned or processed food has been shown to be of disadvantage.

The B- vitamins should be supplemented, as well as lecithin and pantothenic acid. Magnesium and trace elements like zinc, chromium and selenium have been found to be helpful in cases of autoimmune processes. Detoxification of heavy metals like lead and mercury should not be forgotten, because these agents are neurotoxic.

The detoxifying-process for heavy metals can be started with chlorella algae, and if necessary, be completed with DMPS or DMSA as we already mentioned in the chapter on chelate therapy.

Osteoporosis and osteomalacia

These two diseases have common traits, but osteoporosis is a lack of bone mass, whereas osteomalacia is a lack of mineralisation of the bones. The causes for these diseases range from a genetic disposition to faulty nutrition with deficiency of vitamin D and calcium to overconsumption of meat with its phosphorus overhang or the inability to absorb nutrients properly. Also hormonal imbalances can play an important role, which can occur in the late menopause with oestrogen deficiency. Cushing's disease with an excess of cortisole or hyperthyroidism with too much thyroxin can also be a reason.

Very important is the fact that lack of exercise weakens muscular strength and the structure of the bones becomes more fragile.

Impaired bone metabolism can also result from side effects of medical treatment with hormone antagonists. This is now standard in prostate cancer treatment with antiandrogenes or LHRH (lutein hormone releasing hormone) agonists, which prevent testosterone production.

In case of breast cancer regimens with anti-oestrogenes or aromatase-inhibitors now belong to the orthodox standard therapy for every case that is more advanced. This can also enhance osteoporosis.

Faulty nutrition can lead to acidosis thus causing mineral losses. In a state of acidosis calcium and magnesium are not absorbed properly, and they are not incorporated into the bones the way they should be. As both minerals are essential for bone structure, acidosis is one of the major hazards for the health of our bones. To counteract acidosis minerals and vegetables should be present in healthy nutrition, and that is not too difficult to accomplish. Foods rich in minerals such as whole grains and seeds, nuts and vegetables, fruit and milk products can be the main food source. In addition home-made sour milk products and cottage cheese, could be the basis for a rich variety of tasty foods.

Faulty nutrition can become a severe problem for bone metabolism. Therefore acid-forming foods should be avoided, as there are: sugar and white flour products, and also meat and fat in abundance.

Plenty of vegetables as well as the supplementation of minerals will help to keep the metabolism in balance. They should be given together with trace elements, which act as antagonists to toxic heavy metals, which can also impede bone metabolism.

Physical exercise is necessary to build up muscle strength, and thus we also get better bone structure, as bones will dwindle when they are not used and trained with muscle action. Swimming and riding a bicycle is preferable to jogging, especially for people with signs of osteoarthritis, as this way less weight is put on the joints.

For the spine on the other hand working with weights can be essential, as the spine needs some pressure in the direction of the body axis by some weight that is lifted overhead. The weights need not be very heavy, even a few kilograms can make a lot of difference for people who are used to sitting with a hunchback. By training to lift those weights they gradually become more upright. Another important factor for the absorption of calcium is vitamin D, the role of which should not be underestimated. It is not a vitamin in a strict sense, as it can be synthesized in our body through the influence of UV in sunlight.

But nevertheless lack of vitamin D can become a problem, especially in countries with a long winter season.

In our kidneys vitamin D is transformed into the active form called calcitriol, which is necessary for many functions such as proliferation, differentiation and apoptosis of cells. Therefore this vitamin got into the focus of cancer research in recent years. It also plays a role in neuromuscular connection and seems to be able to keep autoimmune inflammation at a low level. Calcitriol also became of interest in the treatment of multiple sclerosis, where blood levels have been found to be low.

This interesting substance calcitriol is essential for the absorption of calcium, and that can become a problem in northern countries. During the winter months with little sunshine the production of calcitriol can be insufficient, and therefore it should be substituted in those cases.

Women after menopause are the main group endangered by osteoporosis, who will profit most from vitamin D substitution. Normally it will be given together with Calcium to make sure they can act together.

There are also natural sources of vitamin D such as fish liver oil or butter, but the fact remains that vitamin D deficiency is quite frequent, especially in women.

The approach to bone diseases from the standpoint of Chinese medicine is different, as energy deficiencies are the most important factor. The kidney energy, especially, should be strengthened, as the bones are ruled by that organ.

There are a number of herbal formulas to help building up new energy for the kidneys and bones. A list of which will be given later.

In homeopathic treatment bone metabolism can be enhanced by several calcium containing substances such as calcium phosphoricum, calcium fluoratum or silica-containing remedies like calcium silicicum.

As also magnesium is an essential part of our bones, it should not be forgotten, therefore magnesium phosphoricum in homoeopathic preparations could be given. Combination with other forms of concentrated magnesium, especially magnesium orotate has been proven valuable, not only for the bones, but also as a remedy against tachycardia and for the soothing of nervous people.

Parkinson's disease

Parkinson's disease belongs to the neurodegenerative illnesses, and is characterised by the deficiency of the neurotransmitter dopamine, which is produced in the substantia nigra of the mid brain. Most prominent symptoms are shaking, rigidity and slow impaired movements, in later phases even dementia can occur.

The therapy in orthodox medicine will either replace the missing dopamine, or apply so-called dopamine agonists. They can bind to dopa-receptors in the brain and enhance the action of dopamine.

All the current remedies have considerable side effects, so that patients often ask for alternatives. Therefore we will consider the treatment from the standpoint of Chinese medicine.

The Chinese view of that disease sees the weakness in the nervous system. Therefore it is important to strengthen the energies pertaining to the nerves, which again is the kidney energy. Several formulas containing Rehmannia would be a way of treatment, as shown in our list of formulas..

Though the illness is not curable, patients feel better with Chinese herbs as a complementary procedure, but we could never replace the orthodox medication completely.

Though there is a hereditary component to that illness, psychological factors such as working in highly competitive positions under a lot of stress or being under pressure from private problems seem to have a part in the development of this deficiency disease.

The restless leg syndrome that keeps patients from sleeping at night, because their legs are constantly twitching, is also caused by a lack of dopamine, and it can be a preliminary phase to Parkinson's. So the orthodox treatment of both diseases is aiming at the same purpose to preserve or replace dopamine.

The approach to these two illnesses in Chinese medicine tries to strengthen the inherited kidney energy, which has a tendency to decrease with age. There are several formulas available for that purpose such as Rehmannia 6 or Rehmannia 8, as well as the eight immortal long life pill.

In all those cases the elimination of the stress factors will be essential. Stress inevitably will lead to depletion of energy by activating the cascade of stress hormones and sympathetic activity of the autonomous system.

Pharyngitis

This illness can have different roots, as it only means inflammation of the throat, which is mostly brought about by viruses or bacteria. It can be acute or become chronic. The acute form is very painful, as the tonsils and the mucous membranes are swollen, and so are the surrounding lymph nodes of the neck. Most acute forms are caused by viruses and are usually accompanied by fever and feelings of acute illness. We already mentioned a few viruses that could cause those ailments, as the Epstein Bar virus in mononucleosis, or the Cytomegalovirus as well as the Herpes 6 virus. There are many more, such as the Rhino-virus group, the Respiratory-syncytial virus, or the adeno-virus group. The problem with these is that they do not respond to antibiotic therapy, whereas bacterial infections with Streptococci or Staphylococci can be treated with those substances. Fungi such as Candida can also play a role in this kind of illness, and there are fungistatic medications available for that purpose.

In cases of chronic pharyngitis it becomes more and more difficult to eliminate the underlying agents. Therefore we found it quite helpful to be able to treat those ailments with homeopathy or Chinese medicine, as often a deficiency of the immune system is present.

The homeopathic approach always takes a close look at the symptoms and modalities, under which an illness occurs or gets worse.

The sudden onset of the disease may speak for the remedy Aconitum, whereas the red and hot head of patients points to Belladonna as a treatment. There are various nosodes available to get rid of pharyngitis, and it depends on the modalities, which remedy has to be chosen to accompany the nosode.

There are special forms of the disease, which go along with bronchitis and cough, and they could call for Mercurius preparations as a remedy or the plant Pulmonaria. A more detailed list of homeopathic remedies will be given after the Chinese formulas.

It is mostly quite useful to go onto a short fast, when the body is fighting a virus and has to concentrate on that process. Then it turns out to be helpful not to have to cope with a lot of food, which needs energy for digestion.

The Chinese way on the other hand tries to find out where the weak points are energetically and may start with acupuncture to alleviate the pain. The next step would be to treat the swollen tissues and get rid of the mucus and inflammation with Chinese herbal remedies in order to open the surface and lead out the heat and wind that has intruded.

Sinusitis

The inflammation of mucus membranes in the nose and throat frequently leads to a complication that can become chronic if not treated in a proper way.

Sinusitis due to viral or bacterial infection can start as an acute catarrh. In case of allergies it is the consequence of frequent or permanent swelling of mucus membranes in the nose or the adjacent sinuses. When there is bacterial super-infection on a sinusitis, which started as virus related, the secretion can become purulent and cause severe headaches. All those manifestations can be treated with homeopathy or Chinese medicine very well, not only when they are in an acute phase, but also when the disease has become chronic.

But then it becomes more difficult to get rid of the inflammation.

Antibiotics should not be applied with viral disease, as this illness does not respond to such a regimen. Even if bacteria have settled on top of the virus lesions, an unimpeded immune system can cope with it and eliminate both viruses and bacteria.

There are not many occasions where antibiotics become necessary. It can become necessary when the sinusitis turns into bronchitis with permanent coughing, thus impeding sleep and many other activities. Then it may be expedient to end the inflammation that has been perpetuated by bacteria in the bronchial tract. In case of an impaired immune system we would otherwise risk progression into pneumonia.

This kind of therapy should still be accompanied by herbal remedies to get rid of the mucus and remaining toxins. There are quite a number of homoeopathic remedies, which can be applied for sinusitis. The nosode sinusitis maxillaris or sinusitis frontalis, which is dependant on the main site of the inflammation, have turned out to be useful.

We will now give a short list of possible remedies to show that the therapeutic success depends on the exact selection of remedies, in cases of chronic illness it becomes most important to observe symptoms very carefully.

1. Belladonna is often needed in cases where the infection is accompanied by throbbing pain, and the patient has a red and hot head, this remedy can as well be given for tonsillitis and pharyngitis, if the symptoms fit.

2. Hepar sulfuris is given when the discharge becomes thick and yellow, showing that bacteria have settled on the mucus membranes, this holds also true for bronchitis.

3. Kalium bichromicum is the remedy to loosen up stringy discharge that is hard to remove.

4. Mercurius solubilis can be given if the mucus membranes are severely affected and the patient is in constant pain where even teeth may feel painful.

5. Pulsatilla has thick green discharge, and feels better in fresh air.

6. Spigelia is the remedy when the left side is more painful, it can be used for other predominantly left sided ailments like heart or headache.

There are also various possibilities to treat sinusitis with Chinese herbal formulas, as colds and sinusitis are considered a wind-cold disease. The herbs have to be selected according to the eight principle ways of diagnosis (ba gang) with emphasis on wind and cold. Later in the course of illness wind and hot symptoms are visible when fever has occurred. Then herbs dispelling wind and heat may become necessary such as Asarum, Ledebouriella or combined with Xanthium in the Xanthium and Magnolia Formula.

For this reason important Chinese herbs will be shown in the next chapter and some formulas where these herbs are used will also be listed.

We will look at this list of Chinese herbs in alphabetical order first and then at recipes to strengthen the vital organs.

Chinese herbs for medicinal use

We will give the botanical name, which is derived from Latin or Greek, first, but also the English name and the Chinese version in Pinyin.

1. Achyranthes bidentata

English name: Ox knee
Pinyin name: Niu Xi
Part of the plant used: root (radix)
Meridians influenced: Liver, Kidney
Taste is bitter, sour, nature neutral
As it tonifies the kidneys, it rules over bones and strengthens back and knees,
Moves blood and dampness
For deficient yin with blood heat and rising liver yang; used for headaches, dizziness, nosebleed, painful menses, not to be taken in pregnancy or with spleen deficiency
Used in the Clematis and Stephania Formula and many others.

2. Aconitum carmichaeli

English name: Chinese Aconite
Pinyin name: Fu Zi
As the plant is extremely poisonous, only a preparation of the root is used, so that the toxicity is removed.
Meridians influenced : heart, spleen, kidneys
The nature of this herb is very hot, so it will be used carefully, in states of weakened yang and to expel cold in kidney and spleen.

It is used in the Rehmannia 8 Formula

In homeopathic medicine the European Aconitum napellus, that is another kind of aconite, is used in diluted (potentized) form for illnesses with sudden onset like influenza or high blood pressure.

3. Acorus gramineus
English name: dwarf sedge, sweet flag
Pinyin name: Chang Pu
Parts of plant used: root
Acrid taste, warm nature
Meridians influenced: heart, liver, spleen
Used for poor memory, lack of clarity of thought, anorexia, bloating, ear infections
Used in formulas like cerebral tonic pill

4. Agastache rugosa
English name: Korean mint, Pachouli
Pinyin name: Huo Xiang
Parts of plant: Whole plant used
Acrid aromatic taste, warm nature
Meridians influenced: Lung, spleen, Stomach
Used for diarrhoea with low fever, vomiting, bloating, headache
Used in Agastache Formula

5. Akebia quinata
English name: Chocolate vine, five leaf akebia
Pinyin name: Mu Tong
Parts of plant used: stem (caulis)
The taste is bitter, nature cool
Meridians influenced: heart, small intestine, bladder

Promotes urination and drains the heat from the heart, is good for insomnia, difficult urination, used in Dianthus Formula.

6. Albizzia julibrissin
English name: Persian silk tree
Pinyin name: He Huan Pi
Parts of plant used: bark
Meridians influenced: heart, liver, spleen, lung
Increases blood circulation and calms the spirit, used for better emotional balance, insomnia, fright, nightmares, paranoia; used in the Formula Concha margaritae and Ligustrum

7. Alismatis plantago- aquatica
English name: Mad dog weed
Pinyin name: Ze Xie
Parts of plant used: bulb
Taste sweet, nature cold
Meridians influenced: Kidneys, bladder
Gently promotes urination, alleviates phlegm retention, pelvic infection. Abdominal bloating, kidney stones and diabetic syndrome. Used in Rehmannia 6 and Rehmannia 6 with Anemarrhena and Phellodendron.

8. Alpinia oxyphylla
English name: Black Cardamon
Pinyn name: Yi Zhi Ren
Parts of plant used: fruit
Taste is acrid, nature warm
Meridians influenced: Spleen, Kidneys
Warms Kidneys and Spleen, stops diarrhea, frequent urination, drooling, abdominal pain

Used in Hoelen and Polyporus Formula

9. Anemarrhena asphodeloides
English name: Anemarrhena
Pinyin name: Zhi Mu
Parts of plant used: root
Taste is bitter, nature cold
Meridans influenced: Lung,Stomach, Kidneys
Used for yin-deficiency heat syndromes, is anti-inflammatory, antidepressant.
Formula: Rehmannia 6 with Anemarrhena and Phellodendron

10. Angelica dahurica
English name: A. dahurica
Pinyin name: Bai Zhi
Parts of plant used: root
Taste is acrid, nature warm
Meridians influenced: Lungs, Stomach
For diseases of cold-wind injuries like headache, colds, congested nose
Used in Xanthium and Magnolia Formula

11. Angelica pubescens
English name: A. pubescens
Pinyin name: Du Huo
Parts of plant used: root
Taste is bitter, nature mildly warm
Meridians influenced: Kidneys, Bladder
Helps to treat pain in lower back and legs,
expels wind and cold
Used in Tian Man and in Eucommia Formula

12. Angelica sinensis
English name: A. sinensis
Pinyin name: Tang Gui
Parts of plant used: root
Taste is sweet, acrid, bitter, nature warm
Meridians concerned: Spleen, Kidneys
For Gynaecological ailments, high blood pressure, tonifies blood
Used in Clematis and Stephania Formula and others

13. Armeniacae prunus
English name: Apricot seed
Pinyin name: Xing Ren
Parts of plant used: seeds
Tate is bitter, nature warm
Meridians influenced: Lungs, Large intestine
Relieves cough, moves large intestine
Used in Clematis and Stephania Formula,
Should not be used in high dosage, can be toxic

14. Aquilaria agallocha
English name: Aquilaria
Pinyin name: Chen Xiang
Parts of plant used: stem
Taste is acrid, bitter, nature warm
Meridians influenced: Lung, Stomach, Spleen, Kidneys
Dispels cold, strengthens kidney Qi, helps proper digestion and asthmatic conditions
Used in Leonurus and Achyranthes formula

15. Artemisia annua
English name: sweet wormwood
Pinyin name: Quinghao

Parts of plant used: leaves
Taste is camphor like, nature cool
Meridians influenced: Lungs, Stomach, Spleen, Kidneys
The drug artemisin is used in cases of fever, and has proven to be effective in the treatment of malaria, we use the plant for the treatment of Chlamydia pneumoniae.

16. Artemisia capillaries
English name: Artemisia capillaries
Pinyin name: Yin Chen Hao
Parts of plant used: shoots and leaves
Taste is bitter, acrid, nature cool
Meridians influenced: Spleen, stomach, Liver, gallbladder
Clears damp heat from liver and gallbladder, for nausea, appetite loss, jaundice
Used in Rhubarb and Scutellaria Formula

17. Areca Catechu
English name: Betel husk
Pinyin name: Da Fu Pi
Part of plant used: husk of betel nut
Taste is acrid, nature slightly warm
Meridians influenced: Spleen, Stomach, large intestine, small intestine
As it moves Qi and reduces stagnation, it is used in treating bloating and congestion
For instance in the Agastache Formula

18. Arisaema amurense
English name: Jack in the pulpit
Pinyin name: Tain Nan Xing
Parts of the plant used: root
Taste is bitter, acrid, nature warm

Meridian influenced: Lung, Liver, Spleen
Dries dampness and expels phlegm
Used in the Cerebral tonic pill

19. Asarum Sieboldi
English name: Wild ginger
Pinyin name: Xi Xin
Part of plant used: whole plant
Taste is acrid, nature warm
Meridians influenced: Lung Spleen Kidney
Used in the congestion of sinusitis, as it repels pathogens, alleviates pain due to wind, not in pregnancy, used in Cnidium formula

20. Asparagus Cochinchinensis
English name: Chinese Asparagus
Pinyin name; Tian Mem dong
Part of plant used: root
Taste is sweet, bitter, nature cold
Meridians influenced: Kidney, Lung
Used for its moistening effects like dry cough or dry constipation, in Ginseng and Astragulus Formula

21. Astragalus membranaceus or propinqus
English name: Milk Vetch
Pinyin name: Huang Qi
Part of plant used: root
Taste is sweet, the nature slightly warm
Meridians influenced: Spleen. Lung
Tonifies the spleen, strengthens the body's defence, used in Ginseng and Astragalus formula

22. Atractylodes macrocephalae

English name: white Atractylodes
Pinyin name: Bai Zhu
Part of plant used: root
Taste is bitter, sweet, the nature is warm
Meridians influenced: Spleen, stomach
Tonifies Spleen and benefits Qi, used in Ginseng and Atractylodes Formula

23. Auranti Fructus
English name: Bitter Orange
Pinyin name: Zhi Ke
Part of plant used: dried fruit
Taste is bitter, sour, nature mildly cold
Meridians influenced: Spleen, Stomach
Used in Bupleurum, Inula and Cyperus against bloating

24. Lophatherus gracilis
English name: Bamboo leaf
Pinyin name: Dan Zhu Ye
Part of plant used: Stem and leaves
Taste is sweet, bland, nature cold
Meridians influenced: Heart, Stomach, Bladder, Small intestines
Used for urinary tract infection, bronchitis; in Lonicera and Forsythia formula

25. Biota orientalis
English name: Arbor vitae seeds
Pinyin name: Bai Zi Ren
Part of plant used: seed
Taste is sweet, acrid, nature neutral
Meridians influenced: Heart, Liver, Spleen, large intestine

Nourishes the heart and calms the spirit, used in Ginseng and Zizyphus Formula

26. Bupleurum falcatum
English name: Sickle hare's ear
Pinyin name: Chai Hu
Part of plant used: root
Taste bitter, slightly acrid, nature cool
Meridians influenced: Liver, Gallbladder, Pericardium
Used with colds and chest congestion, liver, Gallbladder, in Bupleurum and Tang Gui formula

27. Arctium Lappae
English name: Burdock fruit
Pinyin name: Niu Bang Zi
Part of plant used: fruit
Taste: acrid, slightly bitter, nature slightly cold
Meridians influenced: Lung, Stomach
Used in the treatment of fever, measles, swollen throat, in Lonicera and Forsythia Formula

28. Amomi fructus
English name: Cardamom seed
Pinyin name: Sha Ren
Part of plant used: Fruit
Taste is acrid, aromatic, the nature is warm
Meridians influenced: Spleen, Stomach, Kidneys
Used for stomach disorders, vomiting, diarrhoea, in Buleurum, Inula and Cyperus Formula.

29. Carthamus tinctorius
English name: Safflower
Pinyin name: Hong Hua

Parts of plant used: flower
Taste acrid, nature warm
Meridian influenced: Heart, Liver
Used for menstrual imbalances and pain,
Used in Pseudoginseng and Dragonblood formula.

30. Chrysanthemum morifolium
English name: Chrysanthemum
Pinyin name: Ju Hua
Parts of plant used: flower
Taste sweet, slightly bitter, nature slightly cold
Meridians influenced: Lung, Liver
Used for headache and fever (wind injuries) in Prunella and
Scutellaria Formula

31. Cimicifuga
English name: Black Cohosh
Pinyin name: Sheng Ma
Parts of plant used: root
Taste is sweet, acrid, slightly bitter, nature cool
Meridians influenced: Lung, Spleen, Stomach
Used against headache and fever, expels exterior wind and
heat, in Cimicifuga, Ginseng and Astragalus Formula

32. Cinnamomi cassia
English name: Cinnamon
Pinyin name: Rou Gui
Parts of plant used: bark
Taste is sweet, acrid, nature hot
Meridians influenced: Kidney, Spleen, Liver, Bladder
Used for diarrhoea and internal coldness in Tian Man and
Eucommia Formula

33. Cistanche deserticola
English name: Desert-broomrape
Pinyin name: Rou Cong Rong
Part of plant used: whole plant
Taste is sweet, sour, salty, nature warm
Meridians influenced: Kidney, large intestine
Tonifies Kidneys and strengthens Yang, weak and cold lower
backpain, infertility
Used in Cerebral Tonic Pills

34. Citrus reticulata
English name: Tangerine peel
Pinyin name: Chen Pi
Part of plant used: fruit, peel
Taste is acrid, bitter, aromatic, nature warm
Meridians influenced: Spleen, Stomach, Lung
Moves Qi and strengthens spleen, used in Citrus and Pinellia
Formula

35. Codonopsis pilosula
English name: Poor man's ginseng
Pinyin name: Dang Shen
Part of plant used: root
Taste is sweet, nature neutral
Meridians influenced: Spleen, Lung
Benefits Qi, tonifies Lungs, used in Tang Gui and Indigo
Formula

36. Coptis sinensis
English name : Chinese Goldthread
Pinyin name: Huang Lian
Part of plant used: root
Taste is bitter, nature cold

Meridians influenced: Heart, Liver, Stomach, Large Intestine
Quells Fire and detoxifies fire poison in high fevers, sore throat, nosebleed, delirium
Used in Tang Gui and Gardenia Formula

37. Coix-Lacrima-Jobi
English name: Job's Tears
Pinyin name: Yi Yi Ren
Part of plant used: seed
Taste is sweet, bland, nature cool
Meridians influenced: Spleen, stomach, Lungs, Large Intestine
Promotes urination, and clears dampness.
Used in Ginseng and Atractylodes Formula

38. Cornus officinalis
English name: Cornelian Cherries
Pinyin name: Shan Zhu yu
Part of plant used: fruit
Taste is sour, nature slightly warm
Meridians influenced: Kidney, Lungs, Liver
Stabilizes Kidney and liver, stops bleeding and excessive sweating
Used in Rehmannia with Anemarrhena and Phellodendron Formula

39. Corydalis ambigua (derived from the Greek name for lark= korydalis)
English name: Corydalis or lark's spur
Pinyin name: Yan Hu Suo
Part of plant used: root
Taste is acrid, bitter, nature warm
Meridians influenced: Liver, Spleen, Stomach, Lung

Invigorates Blood and alleviates pain and cramps, moves Qi
Used in Tang Gui and Indigo Formula.

40. Curcuma
English name: Turmeric
Pinyin name: Jiang Huang
Part of plant used: root
Taste is acrid, bitter, nature warm
Meridians influenced: Spleen, Stomach, Liver
Relieves abdominal, arthritic, traumatic pain, moves Qi and
invigorates blood
Used in Bupleurum, Inula and Cyperus Formula

41. Cuscuta sinensis
English name: Dodder
Pinyin name: Tu Si Zi
Part of plant used: seeds
Taste is acrid, sweet, nature neutral
Meridians influenced: Liver, kidneys
Tonifies kidneys and benefits essence, sore lower back and
knees
Used in Concha Margaritae and Ligustrum Formula

42. Cyperus rotundus
English name: Red nut Sedge
Pinyin name: Shiang Fu
Part of plant used: root
Taste is acrid, slightly bitter, sweet, nature slightly warm
Meridians influenced: Liver, Triple Burner
Circulates Qi, regulates menstruation and alleviates pain
Used in Cyperus and Ligusticum Formula

43. Dioscorea opposita

English name: Chinese Yam
Pinyin name: Shan Yao
Part of plant used: root
Taste is sweet, nature neutral
Meridians influenced: Kidney, Lung, Spleen
Tonifies Spleen, Stomach and Kidneys in Chronic fatigue and diarrhoea
Used in Rehmannia 6 and 8

44. Dipsacus japonica
English name: teasel
Pinyin name: Xu Duan
Part of plant used: root
Taste is bitter, acrid, nature slightly warm
Meridians affected; Liver, Kidney
Tonifies Liver and kidney and strengthens bones
Used in Tang Gui and Indigo Formula

45. Dolichos Lablab
English name; Hyacinth Bean
Pinyin name; Bian Dou
Part of plant used: fruit or whole plant
Taste is sweet, nature neutral
Meridians influenced: Liver, Spleen
Clears summer heat, strengthens spleen, to treat vomiting and diarrhoea
Used in Ginseng and Atractylodes Formula

46. Eclipta prostrata
English name: False Daisy
Pinyin name: Han Lian Cao
Part of plant used: whole plant
Taste is sweet, sour, nature cool

Meridians influenced: Liver, Kidneys
Nourishes and tonifies liver and kidneys, cools blood, stops bleeding, rejuvenating, against dizziness, blurred vision, premature graying of hair, vertigo, back pain, loss of teeth, used in Concha margaritae and Ligustrum Formula

47. Ephedra sinensis
English name: Mormon Tea
Pinyin name: Ma huang
Part of plant used: Twigs and stems
Taste is acrid, bitter, nature warm
Meridians influenced: Lungs. Bladder
Disperses cold, controls wheezing, reduces oedema
Used in the Ma Huang Formula

48. Eucommia ulmoides
English name: Chinese Rubber Tree
Pinyin name: Du zhong
Part of plant used: bark
Taste is sweet, slightly acrid, nature warm
Meridians influenced: Liver, Kidneys
Tonifies Liver and Kidneys and strengthens bones and sinews, speeds regeneration and healing, used in Tian Qi and Eucommia Formula

49. Evodia rutaecarpa
English name; Evodia
Pinyin name: Wu Zhu Yu
Part of plant used: fruit
Taste is acrid, bitter, nature warm
Meridians influenced: Spleen, Stomach, Liver, Kidneys

Disperses cold, alleviates pain, stops vomiting, warms spleen, stops diarrhoea
Used in Ilex and Evodia Formula

50. Forsythia suspensa
English name: Forsythia
Pinyin name: Lian Qiao
Part of plant used: fruit
Taste is bitter, acrid, nature cold
Meridians influenced: Heart, Liver, Gallbladder
Clears heat and poisons, high fever, lymphatic swellings, urinary infections
Used in Lonicera and Forsythia Formula

51. Fritillaria cirrhosa
English name: Fritillaria, American name: Mission Bell
Pinyin name: Chuan Bei Mu
Part of plant used: bulb
Taste is sweet bitter, nature cool
Meridians influenced: Heart, Lungs
Clears heat, transforms phlegm in chronic cough
Used in Apricot seed and Fritillaria Formula

52. Gardenia jasminoides
English name: Gardenia
Pinyin name: Zhi Zi
Part of plant used: fruit
Taste is bitter, nature cold
Meridians influenced: Liver, Lungs, Heart, Gallbladder, Stomach, Triple Warmer
Clears heat and cools blood in bladder infections, jaundice, ulcerations
Used in Tang gui and Gardenia Formula

53. Gastrodia elata
English name: Gastrodia
Pinyin name: Tian Ma
Part of plant used: root
Taste is sweet, nature neutral
Meridians influenced: Liver
Pacifies liver and extinguishes wind, disperses painful obstructions
Used in Leonurus and Achyrantes Formula

54. Gentiana macrophylla
English name: Gentian
Pinyin name: Qin Jiao
Part of plant used: root
Taste is bitter, acrid, nature neutral
Meridians influenced: Liver, Stomach, Gallbladder
Expels wind dampness in treatment of arthritis, jaundice, constipation due to dryness
Used in: Clematis and Stephania Formula

55. Gentiana scabra
English name: Chinese Gentian
Pinyin name: Long Dan Cao
Part of plant used: root
taste is bitter, nature cold
Meridians influenced: Liver, Stomach, Gallbladder, Bladder
This Gentian acts in a similar way as the other one, but even more pacifies liver fire, high blood pressure, conjunctivitis, urinary infection
Used in The Gentiana Formula

56. Zingiberis officinalis
English name: Ginger
Part of plant used: root
Taste is acrid, nature hot
Meridians influenced: Lungs, Stomach, Spleen
Releases exterior and releases cold to treat vomiting and the common cold
Used in Stephania and Astragalus Formula and many others

57. Panax Ginseng
English name: Ginseng
Pinyin name: Ren Shen
Part of plant used: root
Taste is sweet, slightly bitter, nature slightly warm
Meridians influenced: Spleen, Lung, Heart
Tonifies original Qi, strengthens spleen and stomach and generates fluid
Used in Ginseng and Astragalus Formula and many others

58. Haliotidis concha
English name: Abalone shell
Pinyin name: Shi Kue Ming
Part used: Whole shell
Meridians influenced: Liver, Kidneys
Quells fire and causes yang to descend for treatment of high blood pressure, eye problems
Used in Rehmannia and dogwood fruit Formula

59. Inula
English name: Inula
Pinyin name: Xuan Fu Hua
Parts of plant used: Flower
Taste is bitter, acrid, nature slightly warm

Meridians influenced: Lungs, Liver, Stomach, Spleen
Stops vomiting and stops rebellion
Used in Bupleurum, Inula and Cyperus Formula

60. Ledebouriella sesloides
English name: Siler
Pinyin name: Fang Feng
Parts of plant used: root
Taste is acrid, sweet, nature slightly warm
Meridians influenced: Bladder, Liver, Spleen
Expels wind dampness, alleviates pain, for headaches, chills,
swollen, aching joints, painfull diarrhoea
Used in Xanthium and Magnolia Formula and others

61. Ligusticum Wallichium
English name: Ligusticum
Pinyin name: Chuan Xiong
Part of plant used: root
Taste is acrid, nature warm
Meridians influenced: Liver, Gallbladder, Pericardium
Invigorates blood and promotes circulation of Qi, expels
wind and alleviates pain
Used in: Tang Gui four Formula

62. Ligustrum lucidum
English name: Ligustrum
Pinyin name: Nu Zhen Zi
Part of plant used: fruit
Taste is sweet, bitter, nature warm
Meridians influenced: Liver, Kidneys
Nourishes and tonifies Liver and Kidneys for treatment of
knee and back pain, weak eyesight ringing of ears, gray hair
Used in Concha margarita and Ligustrum Formula

63. Lonicera japonica
English name: Honeysuckle
Pinyin name: Jin Yin Hua
Parts of plant used: Flower
Taste is sweet, nature cold
Meridians influenced: Lungs, Stomach, Large intestine
Clears heat and detoxifies fire poison for treatment of heat-related symptoms with burning urine, swollen tonsils, hot diarrhoea, used in Lonicera and Forsythia Formula

64. Loranthus parasiticus
English name Loranthus
Pinyin name: San Ji Sheng
Parts of plant used: Stems
Taste is bitter, sweet, nature neural
Meridians influenced: Liver, Kidneys
Nourishes blood is calming, for high blood pressure and lower back pain
Used in Tian Qi and Eucommia Formula

65. Lycium sinensis
English name: Lycium fruit
Pinyin name: Gou Qi Zi
Part of plant used: Fruit
Taste is sweet, nature neutral
Meridians influenced: Liver, Kidneys
Nourishes and tonifies liver and kidneys, benefits essence and brightens eyes
Used in Cerebral tonic pills

66. Magnetitum
English name: Magnetic Stone
Pinyin name: Ci Shi
Part used: whole stone
Taste is acrid, nature cold
Meridians influenced; Kidneys, Liver
Tranquilizes spirit, pacifies liver, helps kidneys in grasping Qi, for restlessness, convulsions
Used in Rehmannia and magnetitum formula

67. Magnolia officinalis
English name; Magnolia bark
Pinyin name: Hou Po
Parts of plant used: bark
Taste is bitter, aromatic, nature warm
Meridians influenced: Spleen, Stomach, Lung, Large intestine
Transforms dampness and directs rebellious Qi downward for bloating, nausea, indigestion
Used in Bupleurum, Inula and Cyperus Formula

67a. Magnolia officinalis flower
Flower is used for nose ad sinus problems
Used in Xanthium and Magnolia Formula

68. Concha margaritifera
English name: Mother of pearl shell
Pinyin name: Zhen Zu Mu
Parts used: whole shell
Taste is sweet, salty, nature cold
Meridians influenced: Liver, Heart
Pacifies liver, brightens eyes, calms spirit for dizziness, vertigo, cataracts, insomnia
Used in Concha margaritifera and Ligustrum Formula

69. Moutan radix
English name: Moutan or Peony
Pinyin name: Mu Dan Pi
Parts of plant used: root bark
Meridians influenced: Heart, Liver, Kidneys
Clears heat, cools blood for skin eruptions, Appendicitis, Gynecological problems with stasis
Used in Eight immortal long life pill Formula

70. Myrrha
English name: Myrrh Gum
Pinyin name: Mo Yao
Parts of plant used: Gum
Meridians influenced: Heart, Liver
Reduces swelling and alleviates pain, invigorates blood, helps with trauma or internal imbalances
Used in: Minor Bupleurum Formula

71. Nelumbinis Stamen
English name: Lotus Stamen
Parts of plant used: stamen
Meridians influenced: Kidneys, Heart
Taste is sweet astringent, nature neutral
Stabilizes kidneys, treatment of leucorrhoea, incontinence, frequent urination
Used in Hoelen and Polyporus Formula

72. Notopterygium incisum
English name: Notopterygium
Pinyin name: Chiang Huo
Parts of plant used: root
Taste s acrid, bitter, aromatic, nature warm

Meridians influenced: Bladder, Kidneys
Disperses cold alleviates pain, for headaches, joint pain, sinus congestion
Used in Clematis and Stephania Formula

73. Ophiopogon japonicum
English name: Ophiopogon
Pinyin name: Mai Men Dong
Part of plant used: root
Taste is sweet, slightly bitter, nature slightly cold
Meridians influenced: Lungs, Stomach, Heart
Nourishes Yin and clears heat, moistens intestines and lungs for treatment of constipation, dry throat, diabetic imbalance, restlessness, chronic bronchitis
Used in Ginseng and Zizyphus Formula

74. Paeonia lactiflora
English name: white peony
Pinyin name: Bai Shao
Parts of plant used: root
Taste is bitter, sour, nature cool
Meridians influenced: Liver, Spleen
Nourishes blood, activates circulation, pacifies liver, alleviates pain for treating blood imbalances
Used in: Bupleurum and Tang Gui and many others

75. Perilla frutescens
English name: Perilla leaf
Pinyin name: Zi Su Ye
Part of plant used: Leaf
Taste is acrid, aromatic, nature warm
Meridians influenced: Lungs, Spleen
disperses cold, circulates Qi, for digestive disturbances,

belching, sneezing, coughing
Used in Agastache Formula

76. Phellodendron
English name: Phellodendron
Pinyin name: Huang bai
Parts of plant used: bark
Taste is bitter, nature cold
Meridians influenced: Kidneys, bladder
Antiseptic qualities make it useful against pelvic inflammatory disease and most other
Inflammatory conditions like skin or mouth lesions
Used in Xanthium and Magnolia Formula and many others

77. Pinellia ternata
English name: Pinellia
Pinyin name: Ban Xia
Parts of plant used: root
Taste is acrid, nature warm
Meridians influenced: Spleen, stomach
Dries dampness, transforms phlegm, harmonizes stomach and stops vomiting
Used in Citrus and Pinellia Formula

78. Platicodon grandiflorum
English name: Platicodon
Pinyin name: Jie Geng
Parts of plant used: root
Taste is bitter, acrid, nature neutral
Meridians influenced: Lungs, Stomach
Circulates lung Qi and expels phlegm, expels pus from abscesses in lung or throat
Used in: Xanthium and Magnolia Formula

79. Polygala tenuifolia
English name: Polygala
Pinyin name: Yuan Zi
Parts of plant used: root
Taste is bitter, acrid, nature warm
Meridians influenced: Kidneys, Heart, Lungs
Calms spirit, centres mind, tonifies heart Qi, for restlessness and insomnia
Used in Ginseng and Zizyphus Formula

80. Polygonatum multiflorum
English name: Solomon's seal
Pinyin name: He Shou Wu
Parts of plant used: root
Taste is bitter sweet, astringent, nature slightly warm
Meridians influenced: Liver, Kidneys
Tonifies liver and kidneys, nourishes blood and benefits essence, moistens intestines, moves stool, for chronic disease, general weakness
Used in Polygonatum Formula

81. Poria cocos
English name: Poria Hoelen
Pinyin name: Fu Ling
Part of plant used: fungus
Meridians influenced: Heart, Spleen, Lungs
Taste is sweet, bland, nature neutral
Promotes urination and strengthens spleen, transforms phlegm and quiets heart
For poor appetite, fatigue, diarrhoea, bloating, scanty urine
Used in Clematis and Stephania Formula and many others

82. Prunella vulgaris
English name: Selfheal
Pinyin name: Xia Ku Cao
Parts of plant used: Flowering spike
Taste is sweet acrid, bitter, nature slightly cold
Meridians influenced: Liver, Gallbladder, Lungs
Clears liver and brightens eyes, for swollen lymph nodes, goitre, tumours,
Abscesses, high blood pressure and vertigo
Used in Prunella and Scutellaria Formula

83. Pueraria
English name: Kudzu root
Pinyin name: Ge Gen
Parts of plant used; root
Taste is sweet, acrid, nature cool
Meridians influenced: Spleen, Stomach
Clears heat, nourishes fluids, for fever, sore throat, sinus congestion, shoulder and neck tightness
Used in Pueraria Formula

84. Rehmannia glutinosa
English name: Chinese Foxglove
Pinyin name; Sheng Di Huang
Parts of plant used: root
Taste is sweet, bitter, nature cold
Meridians influenced: Liver, Kidney, Heart
Clears heat and cools blood, nourishes Yin and blood for high fever, thirst, irritability, dry stool, lower back pain
Used in Ginseng and Zizyphus Formula

85. Rehmannia glutinosa praeparata
English name: steamed chinese foxglove
Pinyin name: Shu Di Huang
Parts of plant used: root cooked in wine
Taste is sweet, nature warm
Meridians influenced: Liver, Kidneys, Heart
Tonifies blood, nourishes Yin, for palpitations, insomnia, irregular menstruation, night sweating, diabetic syndrome; used in Tang Gui and Gardenia Formula and many others

86. Salvia miltiorrhiza
English name: Salvia
Pinyin name: Dan Shen
Parts of plant used: root
Taste is bitter, nature slightly cold
Meridians influenced: Heart, Pericardium, Liver
Clears heat and soothes irritability or palpitations, for irritability, palpitations, skin sores, menstrual irregularity, endometriosis
Used in Ginseng and Zizyphus

87. Saussurea
English name: Saussurea
Pinyin name: Mu Xiang
Parts of plant used: root
Taste is bitter, acrid, nature warm
Meridians influenced Spleen, Stomach, Large intestine, Liver, gallbladder
Strengthens spleen and moves Qi, for abdominal and chest pain, nausea, vomiting, weak digestion, asthma
Used in Ginseng and Longan Formula

88. Schisandra sinensis
English name: Schisandra
Pinyin name; Wu Wei zi
Parts of plant used: Fruit
Taste is five-fold, contains all five tastes, nature is warm
Meridians influenced: Kidney, Lungs
Retains essence and stops diarrhoea, stops sweating, calms spirit, for insomnia, morning diarrhoea, asthma, diabetes, palpitations
Used in Xanthium and Magnolia Formula and many others

89. Scrophularia ningpoensis
English name: Chinese Figwort
Pinyin name: Xuan Shen
Parts of plant used: root
Taste is bitter, salty, nature cold
Meridians influenced: Lungs, Stomach, Kidneys
Clears heat, cools blood, nourishes Yin, dissipates nodules, for sore and swollen throat
Swollen eyes, bleeding due to heat and toxicity
Used in Ginseng and Zizphus Formula

90. Scutellaria baicalensis
English name: Scullcap
Pinyin name: Huang Qin
Part of plant used: root
Taste is bitter, nature cold
Meridians influenced: Heart, Lungs, Gallbladder, Large intestine
Clears heat and quells fire, subdues ascending liver yang, for high blood pressure, irritability, red eyes, gall bladder irritation

91. Sophora japonica
English name: Sophora
Pinyin name: Huai Hua Mi
Parts of plant used: flower
Taste is bitter, nature cool
Meridians influened: Liver, Large intestine
Cools blood, stops bleeding, cools liver, for sore eyes, dizziness, intestinal and uterine
Bleeding, haemorrhoids, high blood pressure
Used in Prunella and Scutellaria Formula

92. Stephania tetrandra
English name: Stephania
Pinyin name; Han Fang Ji
Parts of plant used: root
Taste is bitter acrid, nature cold
Meridians influenced: Lungs, Spleen
Expels wind dampness, alleviates pain, for oedema in lower half of body, knee swellings
Arthritis, rheumatism, bloating of abdomen
Used in Stephania and Astragalus Formula

93. Tribulus terrestris
English name: Tribulus
Pinyin name: Bai Ji Li
Parts of plant used: fruit
Taste is acrid, bitter, nature warm
Meridians influenced: Liver, Lungs
Extinguishes wind, alleviates pain, brightens the eyes, for headaches, eye problems,
Itching, Conjunctivitis, nervousness, high blood pressure
Used in Rehmannia and Dogwood fruit Formula

94. Uncaria
English name: Gambir
Pinyin name; Gou Teng
Parts of plant used: Stems and Thorns
Taste is sweet, nature cool
Meridians influenced: Liver, Heart
Extinguishes wind, alleviates spasms, quells heat and pacifies liver, for headaches,
Red eyes, irritability, dizziness, tremors, seizures
Used in Leonurus and Achyrantes Formula

95. Xanthium
English name: Cocklebur
Pinyin name; Can Er Zi
Parts of plant used: fruit
Taste is sweet, slightly bitter, nature warm
Meridians influenced: Liver, Lungs
Disperses wind, expels dampness, opens nasal passages, for headaches, sinus discharge and pain, arthritis, skin disorders, itching, lumbago
Used in Xanthium and Magnolia Formula

96. Zizyphus jujuba
English name: Red date
Pinyin name: Da Zao
Parts of plant used: fruit
Taste is sweet, nature warm
Meridians influenced: Spleen, Stomach
Nourishes spleen, tonifies stomach, moistens dryness and calms spirit, for weak digestion insomnia, hysteria
Used in Stephania and Astragalus Formula and many others

97. Zizyphus spinosa
English name: sour date
Pinyn name: Suan Zao Ren
Parts of plant used: seed
Taste is sour, sweet, nature neutral
Meridians influenced: Heart, Spleen, Gall bladder
Nourishes heart and liver, calms spirit, for irritability, insomnia, palpitations
Used in Ginseng and Zizyphus Formula

Chinese Formulas in detail

1. Agastache Formula for gastrointestinal disturbances with headache, fever, nausea, vomiting, chills, diarrhoea consists of the following herbs:
Agastache, Huo Xiang
Perilla, Zi Su Ye
Angelica sinensis, Bai Zhi
Poria, Fu ling
Pinellia, Ban Xia
Citrus, Chen Pi
Liquorice root, Gan Cao
Ginger root, Sheng Jiang
Atractylodes root, Bai Zhu
Magnolia bark, Huo Po
Areca husk, Da Fu Pi
Platycodon root, Jie Geng

2. Rehmannia with Anemarrhena and Phellodendron for bladder infections, menopausal hot flashes, night sweats, lower back pain contains the following herbs:
Rehmannia prep, Shu di huang
Alisma root, Ze Xie
Cornus fruit, Shan Zhu Yu
Moutan root, Mu Dan Pi
Dioscorea root, Shan Yao
Poria, Fu Ling
Phellodendron bar, Huang Bai
Anemarrhena root, Zhi Mu

3. Angelica Formula for chronic blood deficiencies after trauma or childbirth, Fatigue, menstrual cramps:
Angelica sinensis, Tang Gui
Ligusticum root, Chuan Xiong
Atractylodes root, Bai Zhu
Zizyphi fruit, Da Zao

4. Apricot seed and Fritillaria Formula for coughs with thick phlegm:
Fritillaria bulb, Chuan Bei Mu
Apricot seed, Xing Ren
Snake gall trio, San She Dan
This is often combined with other formulas that treat asthma and bronchitis, also without snake gall trio

5. Bupleurum, Inula and Cyperus Formula for belching, bloating and fullness:
Bupleurum, Chai Hu
Peonia alba, Bai Shao
Citrus, Cheng Pi
Cyperus, Chiang Fu
Auranti fructus, Zhi Ke
Magnolia bark, Huo Po
Cardamon seed, Sha Ren
Citri immaturi, Qing Pi
Corydalis, Yan Hu Suo
Moutan, Mou Dan Pi
Inula flower, Xuan Fu Hua
Liquorice root, Gan cao
Curcuma rhizoma, Jiang Huang
Aquilaria, Chen Xiang
Cardamon seed, Bai Dou Kou
Sandalwood, Tan Xiang

6. Bupleurum and Tang Gui Formula strengthens spleen, nourishes blood, restores harmony between spleen and stomach:
Bupleurum root, Chai Hu
Angelica sinensis, Tang Gui
Paeonia alba, Bai Shao
Atractylodes, Bai Zhu
Poria, Fu ling
Peppermint leaf, Bo He
Liquorice root, Gan Cao
Ginger root, Sheng Jiang Pi

7. Cerebral Tonic Pill for internal dampness that interferes with thought, poor concentration and memory:
Schisandra fruit, Wu Wei Zi
Zizyphus seeds, Suan Zao Ren
Cistanches stem, Rou Cong Rong
Lycium fruit, Gou Qi Zi
Walnut, Hu Tao Ren
Biota seeds, Bai Zi Ren
Acorus rhizoma, Chang Pu
Arisaema tuber, Tian Nan Xing
Amber, resin, Hu Po
Gastrodia rhizoma, Tian Ma
Dragon teeth, Long Chi
Polygala, Yuan Zhi

8. Citrus and Pinellia Formula harmonizes spleen and stomach, dispels congestion in stomach, lungs or sinuses, for general dampness, poor metabolism
Pinellia rhizoma, Ban Xia
Poria, Fu Ling
Citrus, Chen Pi
Liquorice, Gan Cao
Ginger, Cheng Jiang Pi

9. Clematis and Stephania Formula treats symptoms of wind dampness and wind chill, unblocks channels, for gout, sciatica, lower back pain, arthritis of knees and ankles, high blood pressure
Angelica sinensis, Tang Gui
Paeonia alba, Bai Shao
Ligusticum rhizoma, Chuan Xiong

Rehmannia root, Sheng di Huang
Persica pit, Tao Ren
Poria, Fu Ling
Atractylodes alba, Bai Zhu
Citrus peel, Chen Pi
Notopterygium, Qiang Huo
Angelica root, Bai Zhi
Clematis, Wei Ling Xian
Stephania, Han Fang Ji
Gentiana scabra, Long Dan Zao
Ledebouriella, Fang Feng
Achyranthes, Niu Xi
Ginger, Sheng Jiang
Liquorice, Gan Cao

10. Corydalis Formula for pain due to spasm and   cramping, bronchial   spasms, bladder or gall- bladder pain and spasms, dysmenorrhoea, intestinal cramping
Corydalis rhizoma, Yan Hu Suo
Paeonia alba, Bai Shao
Liquorice root, Gan Cao

11. Eight Immortal Long Life Pill
For chronic weakness with thirst, sweating, lower back pain with weak knees
Rehmannia preparata, Shu Di Huang
Alisma rhizoma, Ze Xie
Cornus fruit, Shan Zhu Yu
Moutan cortex, Mu Dan Pi
Dioscorea root, Shan Yao
Poria, Fu Ling
Ophiopogon, Mai Men Dong
Schisandra fruit, Wu Wei Zi

12. Fritillaria extract Formula
For bronchitis with cough, asthma in children
Fritillaria, Chuan Bei Mu
Polygala root, Yuan Zhi
Schisandra, Wu Wei Zi
Platycodon root, Ji Geng
Citrus peel, Chen pi
Liquorice root, Gan Cao

13. Ginseng and Astragalus Formula
For fatigue with fever and poor appetite, strengthens digestive functions
Ginseng root, Ren Shen
Astragalus root, Huang Qi
Liquorice root, Gan Cao
Atractylodes rhizoma, Bai Zhu
Angelica sin. root, Tang Gui
Ginger root, Sheng jiang Pi
Zizyphus fruit, Da Zao
Citrus peel, Chen Pi
Bupleurum root, Chai Hu
Cimicifuga root, Sheng Ma

14. Ginseng and Tang Gui Formula
For Fatigue, chills, gastrointestinal weakness, palpitations, anxiety, after surgery
Ginseng, Ren Shen
Astragalus, Huang Qi
Peonea alba, Bai Shao
Atractylodes rhizoma, Bai Zhu
Poria, Fu Ling

Rehmannia preparata, Shu Di Huang
Angelica sin. root, Tang Gui
Cinnamon root, Rou Gui
Ligusticum root, Chuan Xiong

15. Leonurus and Achyranthes Formula
For high blood pressure associated with central nervous system disorders such as headache, vertigo, numbness
Leonurus seeds, Yi Mu Cao
Coptis rhizoma, Huang Lian
Uncaria, Gou Teng
Amber resin, Hu Po
Angelica sinensis, Tang Gui
Aquilaria wood, Chen Xiang
Ligusticum rhizoma, Chuan Xiong
Gastrodia rhizoma, Tian Ma
Rhubarb rhizoma, Da Huang
Rehmannia root, Sheng Di Huang
Gelatine skin, E Jiao
Prunella spike, Xia Ku Cao
Mutan root bark, Mu Dan Pi
Achyranthes, Niu Xi

16. Lonicera and Forsythia Formula
For symptoms of common cold with swollen lymph nodes, joint aches, headache, sore throat, rashes and hives, relieves wind heat symptoms
Lonicera, Jin Yin Hua
Forsythia, Lian Qiao
Platycodon root, Jie Geng
Peppermint leaf, Bo Hu
Bamboo leaf, Dan Zhu Ye
Liquorice root, Gan Cao

Schizonepeta herba, Jing Jie
Soy seeds, Dan Dou Chi
Burdock fruit, Niu Bang Zi

17. Rehmannia six Formula
For night sweats, lower back pain, chronic sore throat, weak
knees, hot palms nourishes kidney and liver yin
Rehmannia preparata, Shu Di Huang
Alisma rhizoma, Zi Xie
Cornus fruit, San Zhu Yu
Moutan root bark, Mu Dan Pi
Dioscorea root, Shan Yao
Poria/Hoelen, Fu Ling

List of important homeopathic remedies

Aconitum napellus: sudden onset of symptoms like infections or cough, symptoms from sudden shock or fever, fear and restlessness, skin red, dry; throat red and swollen, formerly used as poison for dipping arrows, acts very quickly, used according to homeopathic law: similar with similar (similia similibus curentur).

Allium cepa: burning watery eyes, colds with nose and sinus problems, excess mucous from the nose is acidic and makes the surrounding skin burn, sneezing, hayfever and allergies with stuffed up nose and red eyes.

Antimonium tartaricum: chest and lung symptoms, obstructed respiration, shortness of breath with rattling mucous, anxious oppression of the chest better by sitting up and fresh air worse by lying down, damp-cold weather, sour food or milk.

Apis mellifica: swelling of skin and mucous membranes, erysipelas, inflammation of kidneys, pleuritic and pericardial effusion, stinging pain, soreness, intolerance to heat, worse in the afternoon, after touch and pressure, better in open air or with cold water

Arnica: remedy after soft tissue injuries, bursitis, hematoma, blood loss after birth, great weakness, worse by motion, does not want to be touched.

Arsenicum album: burning sensations with heartburn and sore throat, yet improved by heat and better in summer, burning discharges, skin ailments such as dry eczema or psoriasis, shortness of breath, colds tend to go down into the chest, burning eyes, diarrhoea with burning pain, first remedy after food poisoning; great anxiousness and restlessness, filled with fear.

Belladonna: pain comes suddenly, high fever, red, hot head, great irritability, naughty kids that spit others in the face, swollen lymph nodes, vertigo when turning in bed, worse teething, having a wet cold head, headache after haircut as a peculiar symptom.

Bryonia: dry mucous membranes with thirst, stinging pains with motion, better by pressure, cough is painful, holds chest with both hands, is afraid of poverty or being poisoned, great irritability while sweating, moody worse from motion, being touched, with physical exertion, in warm rooms or hot weather better lying on aching side, by pressure on aching part and cold water to drink.

Calcarea phosphorica: helps with all problems around bones and teeth, such as tooth decay, broken bones; painful joints, numbness in extremities, headaches, better in warm weather and in summer, worse in cold weather, with stress and mental exertion

Cantharis: good remedy for bladder infection with burning hot pain and constant urge, unquenchable thirst with aversion to fluids, restlessness, constantly in motion, burning after insect stings, blood in urine or any other orifice.

Carbo vegetabilis: (vegetable charcoal): good remedy for indigestion, gas in stomach, bloating, belching, skin clammy blue, weakness or collapse with cold limbs, irritable, indifferent to other people better by passing gas, in cold air, worse eating too much especially fatty foods, drinking too much wine and coffee

Chamomilla: for whiny, irritable kids if restless by teething, colic or earache, swollen lymph nodes, fever with one cheek red, the other pale better from being carried around, cold applications worse when in pain, which is unbearable, at night, with wind blowing.

Ferrum phosphoricum: helps to speed recovery after surgery, for inflammation, congestion, fevers that do not respond to Belladonna, restlessness, rapid pulse, throbbing pain in ears, bleeding from nose or other orifices, sore throat, tickling cough, bad sleep with anxious dreams

Gelsemium: onset is slow and gradual unlike aconite and belladonna, flu with body aches, neck shoulder sore, dull headache, running nose, vertigo, dizziness, heavy eyelids, better by bending forward, worse through change of weather, mental exertion.

Hepar sulphur: for unhealthy skin conditions, acne, eczema, foul smelling pus from eruptions, skin sensitive to touch; cough, sore throat with splinter feeling, earache with discharge, swollen lymph nodes, hay fever with itching eyes and throat, feeling chilly, oversensitive, irritable; digestive problems with smelly stool, better from wet warm weather, wrapping ears and head, after eating, worse from lying on painful side and touch, dry cold air, cold food and drink.

Hypericum: (St. John's Wort): pain relief for injuries to areas rich in nerve endings, radiates from the injury, tearing, stiching pains, spinal cord irritation, crushed fingers, burns, hypersensitivity to pain; mental nerve remedy, depression, irritability, stress and shock, better bending head back, worse from touch, fog, cold

Ledum palustre: for bites and stings, pain extends upward, black eye by a blow, rheumatism with pain beginning in feet travels upward, soles and heels sore, gout in big toe, tendency to easy sprains, better from cold application, worse from heat, warm application

Magnesium phosphoricum: abdomen cramping, spasmodic, much belching, sharp, cutting, shooting pain also with menstruation, feeling of constriction, muscle cramps in legs, fingers, better from warmth, gentle pressure, bending double, worse from cold air, draft, cold water

Mercurius vivus: weakness and trembling, sweating, sore throat, gums swollen bleed easily, tonsillitis, earache, swollen lymph nodes, thick nasal discharge, bad breath, teeth loose and tender, slimy bloody stool, straining, cystitis with urging and burning, better when resting, worse heat and cold, during perspiration.

Nux vomica: helps with nausea, belching, sour burping, bloating after meals, heartburn and indigestion after rich foods, overeating, irritability, mental stress from overworking, headache like a nail driven in, itching hemorrhoids, sore throat, running nose, dry cough, insomnia after mental strain and after 3am, better pressure, eating, warmth, rest, worse with mental exertion, anger, coffee, thunderstorm.

Phosphorus: made from phosphorus in bone ash,
major respiratory remedy for deep cough and bronchitis, pneumonia, hemorrhage, anxious, appears less ill than really is, nosebleed, right sided complaints laryngitis, burning pain in stomach, sour taste, belching, vomiting, regurgitation, morning diarrhea of old people, better open air, worse lying on painful side, mental exertion, thunderstorms, getting wet, touch, appears thirstless.

Pulsatilla: (windflower): gentle easily brought to tears, rapid change in mood, many female complaints such as varicose veins, cystitis, edema, overweight, menstrual disorders, depression (better with sympathy), colds, cough, earache with yellow discharge, styes on upper lid, averse to fat food, dry mouth without thirst, bitter taste, flatulence, heartburn, better from open air, cold applications, motion, worse from warmth, lying on left side

Rhus toxicodendron: for back aches, body aches, lumbago after lifting heavy loads, sprains, rheumatism, flu with muscle ache, skin ailments with itchy red spots, fever blisters, shingles, chicken pox, better with movement, therefore restlessness, warm, dry weather, worse in the morning, cold damp weather, overexertion

Ruta graveolens: soreness in the bones, joints, tendons, cartilage, sciatica from sprains, bruises, injuries that are not healing well, dental problems, eye strain from overuse or computer work followed by headache, better lying on back, motion, worse by cold, wet weather, overexertion

Spongia tosta: breathing difficult from cough, croup, asthma, wheezing with persistent mucous, laryngitis with burning sensation, constriction, dry throat, better from lying with head down, worse from wind, talking, exertion, lying down

Sulphur: remedy for red, dirty looking skin, dry eczema, hot, scaly, burning, itchy, acne, with irritated skin, red orifices, eye problems, inflammation of the cornea, conjunctivitis, styes, nausea, constipation, hemorrhoids, better from dry warm weather, lying on right side, standing, worse with heat application, sweating, in open air, milk disagrees.

Veratrum album: sudden shock or collapse, cold sweat, vomiting diarrhea, headache with weakness, hoarse, weak voice, rattling in chest, cramping in calves, painful menses with coldness, better warmth, walking, covering, worse cold weather, lying down, least motion, during stool

Thuja: it acts on skin, gasto-inestinal tract, genito-urinary tract, kidneys and brain, against warts, condylomata, naevi, spongy tumours and damages after vaccination, tearing in muscles and joints, better in dry weather, worse in cold damp weather.

Selected homeopathic remedies for certain indications

Allergies with stuffed up nose, burning eyes, sneezing and coughing

Euphrasia D6 is the remedy for burning and itching eyes as globuli or tablets, also for local application as drops, rinsing the eyes with Euphrasia tea is helpful in case of inflammation.

Cardiospermum D6 for respiratory problems due to allergies or skin trouble with itching and burning.

Galphimia glauca D6 good remedy for sneezing and itching of the nose.

Luffa operculata D6-D12 stuffed up nose.

Apis D6 conjunctivitis with swollen eyelids.

Urtica urens for itching and burning skin or mucus membranes.

Calcarea carbonica D6 for chronic eczema.

Allium cepa D4-D6 for watering eyes and stuffed up nose.

Sulphur D30 for dry Eczema, acne, itching.

Remedies for joint ache, arthritis, rheumatism

Arnica has pains due to bruising

Bryonia D4-D6 is worse with motion, accompanied by swelling

Causticum has jaw and neck pain due to osteoarthritis.

Gelsemium has aching in muscles, headaches often accompanying virus infections.

Rhus toxicodendron shows rheumatic ailments with swelling and stiffness, worse in cold and damp weather, getting better by warmth and motion.

Ruta graveolens heals injuries to bones and stitching with sharp tools.

Remedies for fever, sore throat, lymph swelling, sinus trouble

Aconitum napellus is a good remedy for sudden onset of symptoms such as fever, influenza, high blood pressure.

Apis has pain with intense swelling of mucous membranes and lymph nodes, gets better from cold drinks.

Arsenicum album has burning pain in throat and nose with accompanying chill, craves warmth, lives in a state of fear.

Belladonna is a good remedy if the head is hot and red with fever, dizziness, delirium.

Bryonia is for dry mucous membranes with stitching pain, inflammation of various membranes such as synovia of joints, better not moving.

Gelsemium has headaches in the course of head and throat infections.

Hepar sulphuris has a very sore throat with swollen lymph nodes, splinter feeling, white matter or pus forming on tonsils.

Lachesis muta has pain that starts on left side or is worse there, clothing or pressure on neck causes discomfort, tongue swollen bluish, stitches in heart region.

Mercurius solubilis is a good remedy when the throat is dry, sore and painful, pain worse at night, swollen tongue, bad breath, white matter or pus forming on tonsils.

Phytolacca decandra tongue and mucous membranes are dark red, throat pain is worse swallowing, shooting up to the ears, whole body aches.

Rhus toxicodendron pain gets better by warmth, swelling and itching of mucous membranes.

Remedies for bronchitis, asthma

Cuprum aceticum for spasmodic coughing, asthma.

Kalium bichromicum for tenacious mucous.

Rumex crispus for chronic bronchitis with intense coughing.

Spongia tosta for Asthma, bronchitis.

Gynecological problems

Borax is a remedy if there is white discharge and sore mucous membranes.

Calcarea carbonica has thick discharge with intense itching, lymph swelling, gets worse before menses.

Graphites refers mostly to overweight women with white and acrid discharge.

Hydrastis has stringy discharge with intense itching, inflammation in the whole pelvic region like interstitial cystitis.

Kreosotum acrid discharge with itching and burning, worse standing.

Pulsatilla creamy discharge with soreness, feels better in open air, moody state of mind, feels close to tears.

Sepia has white, offensive discharge with itching and burning, downward pressure and heaviness, irritability.

Lilium tigrinum can help with menstrual irregularities and bladder problems.

Viburnum opulus is a remedy against strong menstrual bleeding.

Cystitis

Cantharis is the best remedy for acute cystitis with cutting and burning pain during urination, it is also called the Spanish fly, but actually it is a small beetle.

Berberis pain goes from bladder to abdomen, this remedy also helps kidneys and Mucous membranes in other locations.

Causticum deep seated pain with involuntary urination on coughing and sneezing.

Nux vomica has constant urging due to irritability of mucous membranes.

Sarsaparilla has urging and burning, weakness of kidneys.

Remedies for liver ailments

Carduus marianus (milk thistle) detoxifies the liver in case of jaundice, nausea, vomiting, headaches.

Chelidonium for sharp stitching pain on the right side with extension to the right shoulder blade, enhances gall flux.

Lycopodium clavatum (clubmoss spores) has bloating and constipation, headache, skin problems, persistent fatigue, dread of failure, insecurity.
Nux vomica for enlarged liver with nausea or vomiting, sluggish bowels.

Podophyllum peltatum relieves congestion and jaundice.

Taraxacum (dandelion) for hardened liver, jaundice, bilious diarrhea.

Recipes for special juices

For type 2 diabetes bitter melon juice has lead to good results, as blood sugar levels could thus be lowered. The juice of one bitter melon slice of about 200 grams should be diluted with a glass of water and drunk slowly within an hour, best be done in the morning.

For people who want to lose weight a special green drink can be recommended with apples, cucumbers, zucchini, celery, broccoli, lemon and ginger.
One medium size cucumber, two celery stalks, two small zucchini, 200 grams of broccoli, one small apple, half a lemon and 10 grams of ginger root is good for 2 persons, otherwise take half the amount if only one person wants to drink it. This drink should be diluted with the same volume of water as you receive from pressing out the vegetables with your juicer.

Açai berries and grapefruit juice

Recently another remedy has been recommended for weight loss, and that is a berry from the rainforest in South America, it is called açai berry and is a powerful antioxidant. But there are too many myths around that berry, and it is not a miracle berry to spare lazy people of motion, if they want to burn more calories in order to lose weight. There are less expensive ways to get a good anti-oxidant, as most of our berries can do almost the same job. Nevertheless açai berries are a valuable antioxidant.

Grapefruit juice is considered valuable, but as it contains furanocumarin derivatives, which interfere with the intestinal enzyme cytochrom P450, decreasing or increasing the bioavailability of a number of drugs, it should be noted, which groups of drugs are concerned.

The group of drugs similar to Valium® (Diazepam) should be kept in mind, as well as

the statin group, such as Atorvastatin (Lipitor®)or

the analgetic or antiphlogistic (pain and inflammation) medication Paracetamol.

There are many more drugs influenced by grapefruit juice, such as carbamazepin, loperamid, omeprazol, codein, nimodipin, L-thyroxin, amiodarone , sertraline, terfenadine, modafinil, astemizol, repaglinide, verapamil and others. People who are under such medication should avoid drinking grapefruit juice.

www.ingramcontent.com/pod-product-compliance
Lightning Source LLC
Chambersburg PA
CBHW070346300526
45791CB00023B/128